£7.95

ABC OF DIABETES

ABC OF DIABETES

THIRD EDITION

PETER J WATKINS MD FRCP

Consultant physician
R D Lawrence Diabetic Department
King's College Hospital, London

with contributions by
P L DRURY, M E EDMONDS

Published by the BMJ Publishing Group
Tavistock Square, London WC1H 9JR

First edition 1983
Second impression 1983
Third impression 1985
Fourth impression 1985
Fifth impression 1987
Second edition 1988
Third edition 1993

ISBN 0 7279 0763 8

Typeset in Great Britain at Apek Typesetters, Nailsea
Printed in Great Britain at the University Press, Cambridge

Contents

INTRODUCTION

Diabetes (literally, a siphon) was known to ancient physicians, but ideas about its causes have evolved over the centuries and still remain uncertain. Since polyuria and wasting are the dominant clinical features—"a melting down of the flesh and limbs into urine" (Aretaeus, 2nd century AD) it was long thought to be due to kidney disease. The discovery of the sweetness of the urine (Thomas Willis, 1621–75) and glycosuria itself (Matthew Dobson, 1776) did not establish the source of the excess glucose. The concept of excessive glucose production was that of Claude Bernard (1813–78), who from his famous piqûre experiments believed that diabetes was due to disease of the central nervous system. These important observations were overshadowed at the time by the demonstration that pancreatectomy caused diabetes (von Mering and Minkowski, Strasbourg, 1889), although Bernard Naunyn (1839–1925), in whose laboratories these experiments were performed, still held that diabetes had its origins both in the central nervous system and in the pancreas. There are undoubtedly many different causes of diabetes: advances in genetics, understanding of the HLA system, and developments in immunology have considerably advanced our understanding of the nature of the disease. Diabetes is a heterogeneous disorder, and even its complications are not uniformly distributed.

The epic discovery of insulin (Frederick Banting and Charles Best) was made in Canada in 1921; the structural formula (Frederick Sanger, 1955) and physical structure (Dorothy Hodgkin, 1969) of insulin were both British discoveries. Innovations in treatment have increased rapidly during the past decade. The outlook for diabetic pregnancy has been transformed; photocoagulation for retinopathy is reducing blindness; and at last diabetic renal disease is receiving some attention.

Underlying much of this work is support from the British Diabetic Association, founded by Dr R D Lawrence and his patient H G Wells in 1934 and now flourishing more strongly than ever. It is an exciting time for diabetic patients and their physicians.

The ABC is intended as a strictly practical guide to the management of diabetes and its complications and is directed to all those doctors and nurses other than established specialists who see diabetic patients.

There have been major developments both in understanding diabetes and its causes and in approaches to management since the second edition. The St Vincent declaration aims to reduce the impact of diabetic complications, while in the UK linking care in hospital with that in general practice, together with the growing effects of audit systems, will improve the quality of care. This third edition incorporates the most important of these innovations.

ACKNOWLEDGEMENTS

Any ideas or inspiration which these pages may contain have inevitably been learnt or borrowed from others. I am indebted to the late Professor J M Malins and Dr M G FitzGerald, through whose enthusiasm I was first introduced to diabetes, and to Dr David Pyke, through whose energy this interest has been fostered over many years. Close collaboration with colleagues at King's has made possible many of the joint ventures described here, and I am grateful to them all. The work of our health visitors, sisters, nurses, chiropodists, dietitians, registrars, and research fellows is the source of constant inspiration. The painstaking work of typing and correcting the manuscript was that of my late wife.

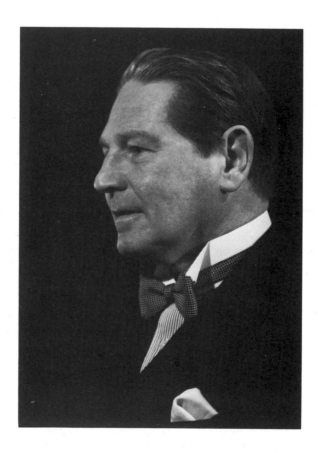

R D Lawrence 1892–1968

Physician, researcher, teacher, and writer, Lawrence was himself diabetic and first received insulin in May 1923. He established the diabetic department at King's College Hospital; played a leading part in founding the British Diabetic Association in 1934, together with his patient H G Wells; and became president of the International Diabetes Federation. In 1925 he first published his famous book *The Diabetic Life*.

WHAT IS DIABETES?

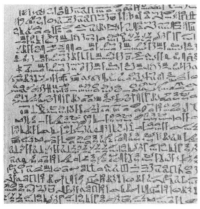

Ebers papyrus: early clinical description of diabetes. (Egyptian, 1500 BC.)

Diabetes occurs either because of a lack of insulin or because of the presence of factors that oppose the action of insulin. The result of insufficient action of insulin is an increase in blood glucose concentration (hyperglycaemia). Many other metabolic abnormalities occur, notably an increase in ketone bodies in the blood when there is a severe lack of insulin.

Diagnosis

	Glucose concentration (mmol/l)		
	Venous whole blood	Capillary whole blood	Venous Plasma
Fasting			
Diagnostic	≥6·7	≥6·7	≥7·8
Uncertain	5·0–6·6	5·0–6·6	6·0–7·7
Random			
Diagnostic	≥10·0	≥11·1	≥11·1
Uncertain	6·7–9·9	7·8–11·0	7·8–11·0

Common mistakes
- Diagnosis and treatment of diabetes on the detection of glycosuria alone
- Diagnosis by blood glucose strip alone—this is not reliable enough to make a lifelong diagnosis
- Requesting a glucose tolerance test when blood glucose concentrations have already confirmed the diagnosis

---

The diagnosis of diabetes must always be established by measuring blood glucose concentration, although glycosuria usually (though not always) indicates diabetes. Criteria for diagnosis are:

- In the presence of classical symptoms—one blood glucose measurement
- In the absence of symptoms—two blood glucose measurements
- In the presence of glycosuria—one blood glucose measurement.

Clearly raised (diagnostic) blood glucose concentrations establish the diagnosis. Where concentrations on two or more occasions are uncertain there are two options:

(1) Glucose tolerance test.
(2) No further action if the patient is elderly and free of symptoms and glycosuria.

Glucose tolerance test

	Glucose concentration (mmol/l)		
	Venous whole blood	Capillary whole blood	Venous plasma
	*Diabetes mellitus**		
Fasting	≥6·7	≥6·7	≥7·8
2 Hours after glucose load	≥10·0	≥11·1	≥11·1
	Impaired glucose tolerance†		
Fasting	<6·7	<6·7	<7·8
2 Hours after glucose load	6·7–10·0	7·8–11·1	7·8–11·1

*In the absence of symptoms at least one additional abnormal blood glucose concentration is needed to confirm clinical diagnosis—for example, 1 hour value of 11 mmol/l or more.
†Patients with impaired glucose tolerance are managed at the discretion of the physician. In general, no treatment is given to elderly people but diet and weight reduction are advisable in younger subjects. Pregnant women with "impaired glucose tolerance" must be treated as if they were diabetic; for interpretation of the test in pregnancy see p 46.

For reliable results a glucose tolerance test should be performed in the morning after an overnight fast with the patient sitting quietly and not smoking; it is also important that the patient should have had normal meals for the past three days and should not have been dieting. False results may also occur if the patient has been ill recently or has had prolonged bed rest. Blood glucose concentrations are measured fasting and then after one and two hours after a drink of 75 g of glucose in 250–350 ml water (in children 1·75 g/kg to a maximum of 75 g), preferably flavoured—for example, with pure lemon juice. Urine tests should be performed before the glucose drink and at one and two hours. Interpretation of blood glucose values according to WHO criteria is shown.

What is diabetes?

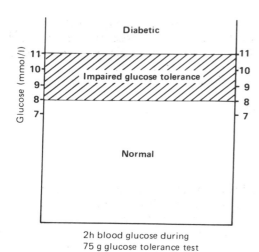

2h blood glucose during
75 g glucose tolerance test

Glucose tolerance tests may also show:

Renal glycosuria, when there is glycosuria but normal blood glucose concentrations; this is a benign condition, only rarely indicating unusual forms of renal disease. It is worth issuing these patients a "certificate" to prevent them from being subjected to repeated glucose tolerance tests at every medical examination.

A steeple or lag curve, when fasting and 2 hour concentrations are normal but those between are high, causing glycosuria; this is also a benign condition, which most commonly occurs after gastrectomy but may occur in healthy people.

Types of diabetes

Diabetes associated with other conditions, and rare syndromes

Pancreatic disease—Pancreatectomy, pancreatitis, haemochromatosis, carcinoma of pancreas, fibrocalculus (calcific) pancreatitis
Hormone induced diabetes—Acromegaly, Cushing's syndrome, phaeochromocytoma, glucagonoma
After burns or other severe illness (Usually temporary, see latent diabetes)
Drug induced diabetes—Corticosteroid drugs and ACTH, especially in large doses; diazoxide. Thiazide diuretics and the contraceptive pill have a weak effect on carbohydrate tolerance
Insulin receptor abnormalities—lipoatrophic diabetes; acanthosis nigricans; antibodies to insulin receptors; abnormalities of the insulin receptor gene
Genetic abnormalities of proinsulin and insulin
Genetic syndromes—(a) Recessive inheritance. Rare families developing insulin dependent diabetes according to a recessive pattern. Other features are associated—namely, diabetes insipidus, optic atrophy causing blindness, and high tone deafness—the DI DM OA D syndrome; (b) Dominantly inherited non-insulin dependent diabetes (Mason-type, see p 3) (c) Other hereditary associations—for example, Prader-Willi syndrome

Although all types of diabetes have hyperglycaemia in common, the causes vary, as does treatment and long term outlook. Nearly all diabetic people have "primary" diabetes, and most of the other syndromes and associations shown in the table are rare.

Primary diabetes mellitus is of two types:
- **Insulin dependent diabetes**
- **Non-insulin dependent diabetes.**

This division is important clinically in assessing the need for treatment and in understanding the causes of diabetes, which are different in the two groups. Nevertheless, although most patients can be clearly distinguished as having one type of diabetes or the other, some non-insulin dependent diabetic people come to need insulin for good health, if not survival; this to some extent blurs the edges of an apparently simple classification.

Other terms
Gestational diabetes—Diabetes which is diagnosed during pregnancy.
Statistical risk classes—Patients with normal glucose tolerance but a substantially increased risk of developing diabetes (a previous or potential abnormality of glucose tolerance).

Insulin dependent diabetes

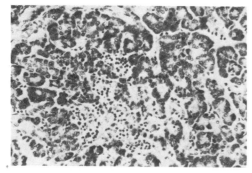

An islet with lymphocytic infiltration (insulitis).

Insulin dependent diabetes is due to damage to and eventual loss of the B cells of the pancreatic islets of Langerhans with resulting loss of insulin production. The agent that damages the islets is not known; in rare cases it may be a virus. The role of autoimmunity is important, thus complement fixing islet cell antibodies develop in genetically susceptible individuals, some of whom become diabetic. More specifically, antibodies to glutamic acid decarboxylase are also found at the onset of diabetes. Not all people with these antibodies develop diabetes, so that at present precise prediction of insulin dependent diabetes in individuals is not possible.

Attempts have been made to prevent the onset of insulin dependent diabetes. Immune suppression with cyclosporin can to some extent preserve islet function, but permanent remissions are not normally achieved and the treatment is in any case too dangerous for routine use. Trials are in progress of drugs which may prevent diabetes by altering macrophage function. Giving insulin itself may conserve islet function.

The incidences of Addison's disease, thyroid disease, and pernicious anaemia are increased in insulin dependent diabetic patients, and appear to occur especially in those with persisting islet cell antibodies.

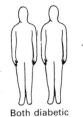

Identical twins

Both diabetic   Non-diabetic Diabetic

Insulin dependent diabetes is not directly inherited, though individuals may inherit a predisposition in that those with certain HLA types show increased susceptibility to this type of diabetes, and almost all are HLA DR3 or DR4; DR2 protects against the development of diabetes. Only about half the pairs of identical twins with insulin dependent diabetes are concordant for diabetes; among the rest one of the pair is diabetic and the other is not.

Non-insulin dependent diabetes

"Mason-type" diabetes

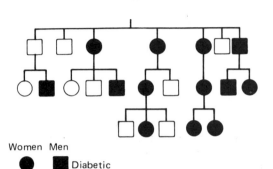

Women Men

● ■ Diabetic

Dominant inheritance of non-insulin dependent diabetes in the Mason family. Several were diagnosed as children.

Insulin dependent	Non-insulin dependent
Inflammatory reaction in islets	No insulitis
Islet B cells destroyed	B cells function
Islet cell antibodies	No islet cell antibodies
HLA related	Not HLA related
Not directly inherited	Strong genetic basis (some cases)

Non-insulin dependent diabetic patients secrete insulin, and their serum insulin concentrations may be diminished, normal, or even increased. Numerous abnormalities, such as inadequate production of insulin, production of genetically aberrant insulins, or peripheral insulin resistance, underly the cause of non-insulin dependent diabetes. The disease has a strong genetic basis: almost all identical twins are concordant for it—that is, both members of the pair are diabetic—and a growing number of genetic aberrations are becoming recognised.

Insulin secretion is reduced in most cases when the patient's weight is taken into consideration. Hyperinsulinaemia may occur in syndromes where there is insulin resistance. Obesity itself is a cause of insulin resistance, and its association with non-insulin dependent diabetes is well known. Women who have had large babies are prone to developing this disease later in life.

Non-insulin dependent diabetes is uncommon in young (under 25 years) white people except in a few families (see below). It is much commoner in black people.

Deposition of amyloid in the islets of patients has recently attracted interest. It is not, however, specific and not always present. Its main constituent is islet amyloid polypeptide, the metabolic effects of which have not been fully elucidated.

There are many well described families in whom non-insulin dependent diabetes is dominantly inherited (Mason-type diabetes); even the children may have the disease. An abnormality of the glucokinase gene has been discovered in some of these families but not in others, and it is likely that other gene defects will be described. Some families may be less prone to the long term complications of diabetes.

Risks of inheriting diabetes

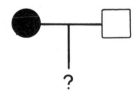

?

A child with a mother with insulin dependent diabetes has an increased risk of developing the same type of diabetes, amounting to 1–2% by 25 years; the risk is about three times greater if the father has this disease. If both parents have it the risk is further increased and genetic counselling should be sought by these rare couples.

Prevalence

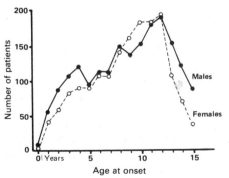

Males

Females

Age of onset of insulin dependent diabetes in 3537 children from the British Diabetic Association register.

In Great Britain 1–2% of the population have diabetes—about half are known to have the condition and the rest can be found by population studies. Among schoolchildren about two in 1000 have diabetes.

Diabetes can occur at any age. Non-insulin dependent diabetes is most common after middle age and occurs most often at 50–70 years of age. The peak incidence of insulin dependent diabetes is at 10–12 years. Nevertheless, elderly people can also be insulin dependent and a few children are non-insulin dependent.

Under 30 years of age there is a slight male predominance of diabetes.

The illustrations of an islet cell is reproduced, by permission of Professor W Gepts, from *Insulin: Islet Pathology, Islet Function, Insulin Treatment*, ed Rolf Luft, published by Nordisk Insulinlaboratorium; that of Mason-type diabetes from Tattersall RB. *Q J Med* 1974;**43**:339–57; and the age of onset chart from *Diabetes in Epidemiological Perspective* edited by J I Mann *et al*, published by Churchill Livingstone 1983.

CLINICAL PRESENTATION: WHY IS DIABETES SO OFTEN MISSED?

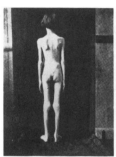
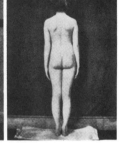

Before insulin   Four months after

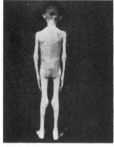
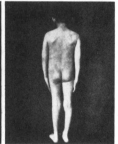

Before insulin   After insulin

Insulin dependent diabetes, 1922.

Thirst, tiredness, pruritus vulvae or balanitis, polyuria, and weight loss are the familiar symptoms of diabetes. Why then is the diagnosis so often missed? Of 15 new patients with diabetes presenting in our diabetic ward for the first time with ketoacidosis, 14 had had no urine test after a total of 41 visits to their doctors. Almost all these serious cases could have been prevented.

Patients do not, of course, always describe their symptoms in the clearest possible terms, or else their complaints may occur only as an indirect consequence of the more common features. Many patients describe dry mouth rather than thirst, and I have seen cases investigated for dysphagia when dehydration was the cause. Frequency is often teated blindly with antibiotics; it may cause enuresis in young people and incontinence in elderly people and the true diagnosis is often overlooked. Complex urological investigations are sometimes performed before the urine is tested.

Confusion in diagnosis

Symptoms of diabetes

- Thirst
- Urinary symptoms
- Pruritus vulvae or balanitis
- Weight loss
- Lethargy

Some diabetic patients present chiefly with weight loss, but even then the diagnosis is sometimes missed, and I have seen two teenagers referred for psychiatric management of anorexia nervosa before admission with ketoacidosis. Perhaps weakness, tiredness, and lethargy, which may be the dominant symptoms, are the most commonly misinterpreted: "tonics" and iron are sometimes given as the symptoms worsen.

Deteriorating vision is not uncommon as a presentation, due either to a change of refraction causing myopia or to the early development of retinopathy. Foot ulceration or sepsis in older patients brings them to accident and emergency departments and is nearly always due to diabetes. Occasionally neuritis is the presenting symptom, causing exquisite pain in the feet, thighs, or trunk.

Glycosuria itself is responsible not only for the monilial overgrowth which causes pruritus vulvae or balanitis; some older men are first aware of diabetes when they notice white spots on their trousers. In hot climates drops of sugary urine attract an interested population of ants, and at least one patient now attending the clinic at King's College Hospital presented in this way before he came to England.

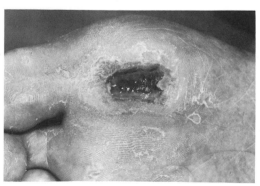

Diabetes may present as a neuropathic foot ulcer.

Patterns of presentation

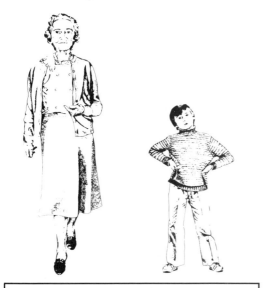

Insulin dependent diabetes occurs not only in young people but also in elderly people

Symptoms are similar in the two types of diabetes (insulin dependent and non-insulin dependent), but they vary in their intensity. The presentation is most typical and the symptoms develop most rapidly in patients with insulin dependent diabetes; they usually develop over some weeks, but the duration may be a few days to a few months. There is usually considerable weight loss and exhaustion. If the diagnosis is missed, diabetic ketoacidosis occurs (see below). Insulin dependent diabetes may occur at any age, even in the very old, but is more common in patients under 30 years of age.

Symptoms in patients with non-insulin dependent diabetes are similar but insidious in their onset; sometimes these patients deny any symptoms, although they often admit to feeling more energetic after treatment has been started. These patients are usually middle-aged or elderly, but children do occasionally develop non-insulin dependent diabetes.

Identifying patients in need of insulin

Symptoms	Age
Rapid onset	Any, more likely under 30
Substantial weight loss	
Weakness	Blood glucose concentration
Vomiting	Any
Signs	Other indications
Usually thin	When tablets have failed
Dry tongue	during pregnancy
Weak	When diet has failed
	during intercurrent illness
Ketoacidosis	In patients who have
Drowsiness	undergone pancreatomy
Dehydration	
Overbreathing	Ill patients need admission
Breath smelling of acetone	Others may start insulin at home
	If there is any doubt *use insulin*

Patients in need of treatment with insulin must be identified. This is done by judging the patient's clinical features: blood glucose concentrations offer a relatively poor guide, although most patients with a blood glucose concentration greater than 25 mmol/l are likely to need insulin.

Features suggesting a need for insulin are: a rapid development of symptoms; substantial weight loss—patients are usually thin, vomiting, and have a dry tongue or more severe dehydration; weakness; and ketoacidosis—these patients are drowsy, dehydrated, overbreathing, and their breath smells of acetone (though many people are unable to detect this smell).

The following groups of patients are likely to need insulin: children and most of those under 30 years of age; women who present during pregnancy; diabetic patients whose tablet treatment has failed; all patients who have undergone pancreatectomy. If there is any doubt give insulin. It can never be wrong to do so, and if the decision was mistaken it can easily be reversed.

Blood glucose and urine tests

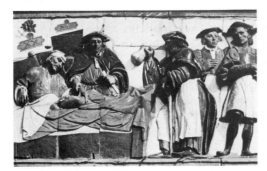

Della Robbia panel from the Ospedale del Ceppo, Pistoia, 1514.

The diagnosis of diabetes should no longer be missed. New patients attending their doctor, whether their family doctor or at a hospital outpatient clinic, should have a blood glucose measurement or at the very least a urine test, especially if their symptoms are unexplained. Only a few diabetic patients are wholly without symptoms and their diabetes is detected by screening at routine medical examinations.

The first illustration is taken from Geyelin H R and Marrop G. *Journal of Metabolic Research* 1922;2:767–91.

TREATMENT

Aims

- Save life
- Alleviate symptoms
- Achieve good control
- Minimise complications

The aims of treatment are, firstly, to save life and alleviate symptoms, and, secondly, to achieve the best possible control of diabetes with blood glucose concentrations maintained as near normal as possible to minimise long term complications. The first aim is relatively easy to attain, and in some elderly patients or those who lack motivation or ability it is the only aim.

	Targets for control		
	Very good*	Acceptable	Less than ideal
Body mass index (kg/m^2)	<25	<27	>27
HbAl₁† (%) (normal 5·0–7·5)	<7·5	7·5–8·8	>8·8 (>10–very poor)
HbA₁c† (%) (normal 4·0–6·0)	<6·0	6·0–7·0	>7·0 (>8–very poor)
Total cholesterol‡ (mmol/l)	<5·2	<6·5	≥6·5
High density lipoprotein cholesterol (mmol/l)	>1·1	>0·9	<0·9
Blood pressure (mm Hg)	<140/90‡	<160/95	>160/95
Blood glucose in non-insulin dependent diabetes§ (mmol/l):			
Fasting	<6·7	<8	≥10
Random	4·0–9·0	<10·0	≥10·0

* This is the ideal and may be difficult, impossible, or unnecessary to achieve in certain patients (for example, elderly people). Individual targets should be established for each patient.
† Reference ranges for HbA₁ vary greatly depending on the method.
‡ Less strict target may be appropriate in older patients; age related charts should be used for younger patients.
§ The optimal range in insulin dependent diabetes is about 4–10 mmol/l (see page 16).

Control is achieved by lowering blood glucose using either diet alone, diet and oral hypoglycaemic agents, or diet and insulin. Patients who need insulin immediately were described in the previous chapter. All others are normally started first on a diet alone, and tablets are added if that fails. The ideal goals are shown in the table.

Other important aims in management include control of weight and elimination of risk factors, notably hypertension, smoking, and hazards to the feet.

Diet

Simple dietary guidelines

- Never take any form of sugar
- Do not take too much fat or carbohydrate
- There is no need to restrict most meat, fish, or vegetables
- Control your weight

There is no need to buy proprietary diabetic foodstuffs. Most forms of alcohol (other than sweet wines and liqueurs) are suitable for diabetics, with the usual restrictions for the overweight

Diet is the cornerstone of diabetic treatment, and control of the diet should always be the first treatment offered to non-insulin dependent patients before drugs are considered. Eliminating sugar (sucrose and glucose) lowers blood glucose concentrations in both insulin dependent and non-insulin dependent patients, and although recent dietary recommendations suggest that eating small amounts of sugar is of little consequence, I do not recommend this practice. Artificial sweeteners can be used. Good dietary advice is essential to the proper care of diabetic patients; ill considered advice can be very damaging or else it is ignored. I recall one patient who kept to the same sample menu for many years before she reported it to be rather boring. Diet needs to be tailored to the patient's age and weight, type of work, race, and religion.

Diets for non-insulin dependent patients

KING'S COLLEGE HOSPITAL—
DIABETIC DEPARTMENT

A DIABETIC DIET

DO NOT EAT OR DRINK:

Sugar or glucose in any form and do not use sugar in your cooking.
Jam, marmalade, honey, syrup or lemon curd.
Sweets or chocolates.
Cakes and sweet biscuits.
Tinned fruit.
Lucozade, Ribena, Coca-Cola, Pepsi-Cola, lemonade and other fizzy drinks.
Apart from these foods and drinks, you may eat and drink anything else, just as you did before you were diabetic.
You may use artificial sweeteners, such as saccharin, Sweetex, Hermesetas, Saxin, but NOT Sucron, and any sugar free drinks including Squashes and Slimline range.
KCH 335

Diets for non-insulin dependent diabetic patients should aim to eliminate all forms of sugar and restrict the total energy intake. Many of the patients are overweight, and their main goal is to lose weight, although this aim is difficult to achieve. It is important to try to ensure that when patients reduce their carbohydrate intake they do not replace it by an increase of fatty foodstuffs, notably a high intake of cheese. The present emphasis is on reducing total calorie intake, with special emphasis on fat reduction and a proportionately more generous allowance of carbohydrate than in previous years. It has been suggested that as much as half the energy content of the diet may be derived from carbohydrates, while the fat intake is drastically reduced, although these diets may in practice require rather difficult and radical changes

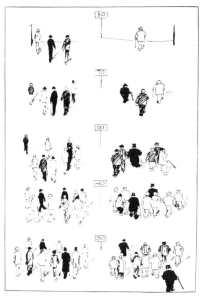

How 10 fat men and 10 lean men fare on the journey through life (Joslin, 1941).

in the types of food normally eaten. The use of polyunsaturated fats is probably desirable, although the debate continues. High fibre diets are of value and may help to reduce blood glucose concentrations if enough fibre is taken. Bran, All Bran, wholemeal bread, and beans have a relatively high fibre content, and are therefore recommended, but foodstuffs with really high fibre content, such as guar gum, are unpalatable.

For some elderly patients it is enough simply to eliminate all forms of sugar from the diet. Their blood glucose concentrations then fall and symptoms resolve. Optimal control may not be needed or even desirable, and it is best to interfere as little as possible with a patient's usual way of life. Dietary advice for these patients can be presented on a postcard.

Diets for insulin dependent patients

Some artificial sweeteners

Aspartame based	Hermesetas Gold
	Canderel
	Sweetex Plus
Saccharin based	Sweetex
	Saxin
	Hermesetas

Sugarlite, Sucron, and Sweetex powders contain sugar and should not be used. Sorbitol and fructose are suitable for baking but high in calories.

The following will increase the fibre content of the diet:

Bread	Wholemeal or stoneground— wholemeal for preference. If these are not available use HiBran or wheatmeal or granary loaves
Biscuits and crispbreads	Ryvita, Macvita, and similar varieties. Digestive, oatcakes, coconut, and bran biscuits, etc. Crackawheat
Breakfast cereals	Porridge, Weetabix, Weetaflakes, All Bran, Bran Buds, Shredded Wheat, Oat Crunchies, muesli, Alpen, and similar cereals
Wholemeal flour or 100% rye flour	Should be used with white flour for making bread, scones, cakes, biscuits, puddings, etc
Fresh fruit and vegetables	Should be included at least twice daily. The skin and peel of fruit and vegetables such as apples, pears, plums, tomatoes, and potatoes should be eaten
Dried fruit and nuts	Eat frequently
Brown rice, wholemeal pasta	
Pulse vegetables	Such as peas and all varieties of beans

Greater finesse is required in managing the diets of insulin dependent patients: if they eat too much, diabetic control deteriorates; if they eat too little they become hypoglycaemic. The important principles are that the carbohydrate intake be steady from day to day and that it should be taken at fairly regular times each day. If this discipline is not followed diabetic control becomes difficult. Severe carbohydrate restriction is not necessarily required; indeed, if the diet is fairly generous patients are less likely to resort to a high fat intake, which may be harmful in the long term.

The actual requirement for carbohydrate varies considerably; it is unsatisfactory to prescribe less than 100 g daily, and control may become more difficult if more than 250 g daily is allowed. The smaller amounts are more suitable for elderly, sedentary patients while the larger amounts are more appropriate for younger, very active people. Although it has been observed that not all carbohydrate containing foodstuffs are equally absorbed and they therefore do not have the same influence on blood glucose values, there is little factual information on this problem and it is impossible to make allowances, other than recommending that sugar (sucrose) should be avoided except for the treatment of hypoglycaemia.

For social convenience it is customary to advise that most of the carbohydrate should be taken at the main meals—breakfast, lunch, and dinner—even though these are not necessarily the times when, according to blood glucose profiles, most carbohydrate is needed; for example, less carbohydrate at breakfast and more at mid-morning and lunch often improves the profile. Snacks should be taken between meals—that is, at elevenses, during the afternoon, and at bedtime—to prevent hypoglycaemia; at least the morning and night snacks are essential and should never be missed.

For convenience 10 g of carbohydrate is described as "one portion," so that a 170 g carbohydrate diet is described to patients as one of "17 portions." Patients need to know the number of carbohydrate portions of different foodstuffs.

Oral hypoglycaemics

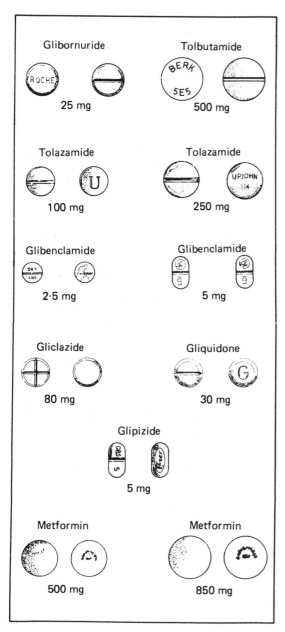

Glibornuride
25 mg

Tolbutamide
500 mg

Tolazamide
100 mg

Tolazamide
250 mg

Glibenclamide
2·5 mg

Glibenclamide
5 mg

Gliclazide
80 mg

Gliquidone
30 mg

Glipizide
5 mg

Metformin
500 mg

Metformin
850 mg

Slightly smaller than life size.

Oral hypoglycaemics should be given only when dietary treatment alone has failed after a proper trial period, usually lasting at least three months. They should not normally be given as the initial treatment (this is a common error).

There are two types of oral hypoglycaemic drugs with entirely different modes of action: sulphonylureas and biguanides. They can be used singly or together. They have an established place in treatment and are used by 30% of all diabetic patients. Unlike insulin, they are not essential for life and should be withdrawn whenever dietary treatment alone will suffice.

Sulphonylureas are generally preferred to biguanides because they are more potent and have fewer side effects. There should be no reluctance to use sulphonylureas even in overweight patients who remain symptomatic despite proper dietary management. A biguanide may occasionally be used as the first line of treatment in grossly obese patients, chiefly because it will help weight reduction to a small extent. Otherwise, a biguanide is generally added to a sulphonylurea if this alone has failed. There are unfortunately many overweight patients who never achieve adequate control, and medical advice is frustratingly of no avail. If a patient remains unwell and continues to lose weight, it is best to switch to insulin without delay. Some patients who just manage to maintain adequate control with maximum doses of oral hypoglycaemics together with a minute diet are extremely grateful when they are changed to insulin and a more generous diet.

Oral hypoglycaemics should not usually be taken during pregnancy. If a diet alone is insufficient then insulin should be given.

Drug interactions are uncommon. Alcohol may dangerously potentiate the hypoglycaemic effect of oral hypoglycaemics. Aspirin, butazolidine, sulphonamides, and monoamine oxidase inhibitors may enhance the hypoglycaemic effect of sulphonylureas, but the hazard is probably small and should not prohibit the use of such drugs if they are needed. Corticosteroids have a powerful hyperglycaemic action, especially in larger doses, and may necessitate a change of treatment to insulin. The indications for their use are, however, the same as in non-diabetic patients, and they should not be withheld just because the patient is diabetic. Thiazide diuretics should be avoided if possible. Oral contraceptives have a weak hyperglycaemic effect but rarely disturb diabetic control.

Sulphonylureas

The hypoglycaemic effect of early sulphonamides was observed in the 1940s, and in the next decade first tolbutamide (1956) and then chlorpropamide (1957) were introduced into clinical practice. They act chiefly by stimulating insulin release from the B cells of the pancreatic islets.

Seven sulphonylureas are available. They are remarkably safe and free from side effects, although rare toxic effects have been reported, including rashes and jaundice. Only one sulphonylurea should be used at a time since there is nothing to be gained from any combination of these drugs and there is no evidence that any one drug is likely to be more successful than another.

Selecting a sulphonylurea is largely a matter of personal choice. Glibenclamide is the most popular; it is taken once or, if larger doses are needed, twice each day. Hypoglycaemia is not rare and is a serious, occasionally fatal, hazard in elderly people and those with renal impairment. In these patients drugs with a shorter half life and which are metabolised before excretion are preferable, and include gliclazide, tolbutamide, and gliquidone. If hypoglycaemia occurs in any patient taking a sulphonylurea the drug should be stopped or at the very least the dose substantially reduced. For the same reason the smallest dose should be used when treatment is started since some patients are extremely sensitive to these drugs.

Chlorpropamide is now obsolete. It has a very long half life, thus increasing the risk of hypoglycaemia, and many patients experience an unpleasant facial flush on drinking very small amounts of alcohol.

	Dose range (mg)
Sulphonylureas:	
Tolbutamide	500–2000
Tolazamide	100–750
Glibenclamide	2·5–15
Glipizide	2·5–30
Glibornuride	12·5–75
Gliclazide	40–320
Gliquidone	15–180
Biguanide:	
Metformin	1000–2000

Biguanides

Biguanides act chiefly by reducing hepatic glucose production. Metformin is now the only biguanide that should be used because phenformin has, albeit rarely, caused fatal lactic acidosis in some patients. This side effect has also been reported with metformin in patients with renal failure or any state of shock: metformin should therefore never be used in these conditions or in elderly patients or those with serious liver disease.

Metformin has several unpleasant side effects, which include nausea, diarrhoea, and vomiting, and may cause a disagreeable metallic taste. Some patients suffer an insidious malaise and are grateful when the drug is withdrawn.

Guar gum

Guar gum preparations, if taken in adequate quantity three times a day before meals, can reduce postprandial blood sugar concentrations. Flatulence is common. There are at present two available preparations—Guarem and Guarina.

Indication for insulin in non-insulin dependent patients

Whether to give insulin to non-insulin dependent patients is one of the most important yet difficult decisions to be made in treating these patients. Failure to give insulin to some patients results in protracted and needless malaise if not actual danger. On the other hand, giving insulin inappropriately can cause needless problems, notably from hypoglycaemia and weight gain. Indications for giving insulin to inadequately controlled non-insulin dependent patients are as follows:

- Insulin is usually contraindicated in overweight patients whose weight is increasing—giving insulin will make this worse
- Patients who continue to lose weight usually need insulin
- Achievement of tight control in order to prevent complications is obviously more important in younger than in older patients, so the patient's age needs to be considered in deciding whether or not to start giving insulin
- Many older patients, however, benefit greatly from insulin treatment, with an improvement of wellbeing, and insulin should not be withheld on grounds of age alone

- Continuing weight loss (even if this is insidious) and persistent symptoms, or both. Insulin treatment in these patients almost always results in a substantial improvement in health
- A non-obese patient without symptoms whose weight is stable and who is conscientious with existing treatment can be given a trial of insulin of about three months' duration. Diabetic control will usually, though not always, improve, and about a half of patients will enjoy a great improvement in health. If this treatment fails to achieve any benefits after about three months the patient has the option to return to treatment with oral hypoglycaemics
- An obese patient without symptoms whose weight is stable presents an even more difficult problem: the correct treatment is intensification of diet, but a few of these patients will benefit from insulin. A three months trial of insulin can be very valuable
- Insulin is often required in patients with intercurrent illness. Many disorders, notably infections, increase insulin resistance, leading to the temporary need for insulin. Withdrawal of insulin after recovery from the illness is important provided adequate control is achieved.

Steroids always exacerbate hyperglycaemia and often precipitate the need for insulin. This should not deter doctors from prescribing steroids when they are needed.

The third illustration, of how 10 fat men and 10 lean men fare on the journey through life, is taken, by permission, from *Diabetic Manual* by Elliott P Joslin, published by Lea and Febiger.

INSULIN TREATMENT

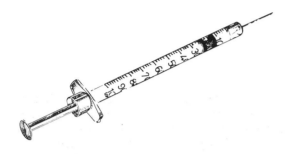

The use of insulin has to be tailored to meet individual requirements. The aim is to achieve the best possible control in the circumstances, avoiding at all costs the disabling hypoglycaemia that can occur if too fine a degree of control is attempted. In elderly patients or those who lack motivation it is therefore wise to aim only at alleviating symptoms and not to attempt very strict control.

Types of insulin

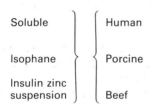

Soluble ⎫⎧ Human

Isophane ⎬⎨ Porcine

Insulin zinc suspension ⎭⎩ Beef

There are three main types of insulin.

Soluble insulins were first introduced in 1922 and still play an important part not only in daily maintenance of insulin dependent patients, but also in managing diabetic emergencies, when they can be given intravenously or intramuscularly.

Protamine insulins are long and medium acting insulins introduced in Denmark during the 1930s.

Insulin zinc suspensions were first introduced during the 1950s; there are several preparations with widely ranging durations of action.

Some preparations of insulin are presented as proprietary mixtures, eliminating the need for patients to mix insulins in the syringe. Details of the types of insulin available in the UK are shown in the table.

Insulin of three species is available: human insulin, manufactured either by modification of porcine insulin (emp) or biosynthetically (crb, prb, or pyr); porcine insulin; and beef insulin. Most patients now receive human insulin. Indications for reverting to porcine insulin in patients with problems caused by hypoglycaemia are described on page 22. Beef insulins are rarely used.

100 U/ml preparations of insulin available in the United Kingdom

Neutral soluble insulins	Isophane insulins	Zinc suspensions	Mixtures (for syringe)*
Velosulin (P or H†)	Insulatard (P or H†)	Monotard (H‡)	Initard (50/50 Velosulin/Insulatard; P or H†)
Actrapid (H‡)	Protaphane (H‡)	Humulin Lente (H‡)	Mixtard (30/70 Velosulin/Insulatard; P or H†)
Humulin S (H‡)	Humulin I (H‡)	Human Ultratard (H‡) Humulin Zn (H‡)	Actraphane (30/70 Actrapid/Protaphane; H‡)

* For other mixtures see table on p 12.
P = Pork insulin.   H† = Human insulin emp (pork modified).   H‡ = Human insulin biosynthetic.
Some other insulins including a few bovine preparations are still available but rarely used.

Selection of insulin

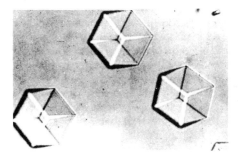

Porcine insulin crystals.

The choice of insulin preparation is based on the duration of action. Although insulins can be broadly classified as having short, medium, or long durations of action, their effect varies considerably from one patient to another: thus soluble insulin, usually considered to be of rather short duration, may have a more sustained effect in one patient than isophane insulin, generally described as a medium acting insulin, has in another patient. The duration of action of insulin in an individual patient can therefore be discovered only by trial and error.

Insulin regimens

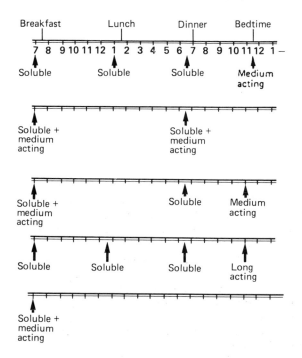

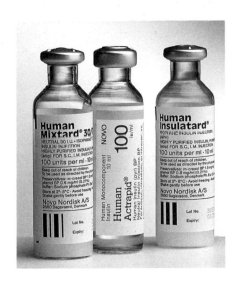

Starting insulin

For relatively ill patients with acute onset diabetes, treatment should be started with short acting soluble insulin two to four times a day. For those less severely ill, treatment should be started with a medium acting insulin or an insulin mixture containing premixed short and medium acting insulins given twice daily; 8 units twice daily is a suitable initial dose for most patients. Many patients who present with acute diabetes enter remission soon after diagnosis, when a small dose of almost any insulin is enough to maintain good control. The practice of withdrawing insulin at this stage is not encouraged because after a few months the need for insulin is almost inevitable.

Maintenance regimens

Most insulin dependent patients who want to achieve very good control will need twice daily injections, but multiple injections (three or four times daily) may improve control, and to some extent increase flexibility (for example, the timing of the midday meal) and are often needed in pregnancy. Multiple injections can be made easier by the use of the insulin in cartridge form administered by apparatus which meters the dose (such as Novo Pen, see page 12). Suitable insulin regimens are as follows.

Twice daily—(1) Premixed soluble and isophane insulins before breakfast and evening meal, or (2) self-mixing short and medium acting insulins or (3) medium acting insulin alone.

Three times daily—(4) Mixture of neutral soluble and medium acting insulins before breakfast; neutral soluble insulin alone before evening meal; medium acting insulin alone before bedtime. This is one of the best insulin regimens if twice daily administration proves inadequate.

Four times daily—(5) Neutral soluble insulin alone before each of the three main meals and medium acting insulin at bedtime. (Occasionally the long acting Human Ultratard insulin is given, though this has not proved to be advantageous.)

There are several suitable medium acting insulins, but those most often used are either one of the isophane preparations or Human Monotard insulin (see table, page 10).

When changing from one insulin regimen to another some trial and error by regular blood glucose monitoring is always needed. In converting a patient to the four times daily regimen the normal dose should be divided by four and a slight adjustment made to give more than one quarter before breakfast and less than one quarter before bedtime.

For some elderly or other dependent patients a single daily injection may suffice, and this has the added advantage of preventing the nocturnal hypoglycaemia, which is a hazard especially for elderly patients living alone.

The availability of pre-mixed insulins in either vials or pen cartridges is a considerable advantage for most patients, especially those who find it difficult to mix insulins in the syringe.

Insulin treatment

Syringes and other devices

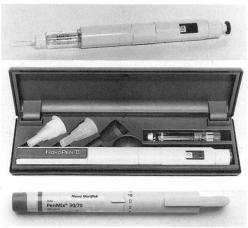

Insulin U100 syringes (BS 1619) are marked directly in units. Most patients should use the 0·5 ml syringe (which takes 50 U), but a 1 ml syringe is available for the few who need 50–100 U in each injection. Disposable syringes are cheap and can be used repeatedly. The best are those with fixed needles; after use the cap should be replaced over the needle and the syringe kept in the refrigerator. Plastic syringes should not be stored in spirit. For blind people a glass syringe is available with a locking screw on the plunger which can be set to deliver a specific dose. Needle size is traditionally 25 G but finer 27 G needles are popular with many patients.

Several insulin "pen" devices deliver metered doses of insulin from an insulin cartridge. They are portable and simplify the procedure of measuring the insulin. Modern pens allow the patient to dial up their required dose and some pens feature both audible and palpable dose graduations to facilitate accurate dosing in patients with impaired vision or hearing, or both. The most recent development in pen technology is a preloaded disposable insulin pen (PenMix 30/70), containing 300 units of insulin. Some insulin pens and cartridges are given in the box. All are human soluble/isophane insulin mixtures (x%/y%), although cartridges containing Actrapid alone are also made.

Pen	Cartridges
NovoPen II (Novo Nordisk)	PenMix Penfills 10/90, 20/80, 30/70,* 40/60, and 50/50*; Human Actrapid; and Protaphane
Becton Dickinson Pen	Humulins M1 (10/90), M2 (20/80), M3 (30/70), and M4 (40/60)
Pur-In Pen* (CP)	Pur-In Mixes 15/85, 25/75, and 50/50
AutoPen (Owen Mumford)	Multidose insulin cartridges

* Also available as vials.

Administration of insulin

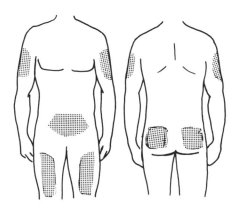

Insulin for routine treatment is given subcutaneously by intermittent injections or by continuous infusion. Insulin can be injected subcutaneously almost anywhere if there is enough flesh. The best site is the front of the thigh. The lower abdominal wall, buttocks, and upper arms may also be used. Women who want to wear short sleeves should normally avoid using the arms in case unsightly marks should appear: some may then prefer to confine injections to the bikini area.

It is important to vary the injection sites from day to day, using, for example, each thigh alternatively over as wide an area as possible. Absorption of insulin varies from one site to another, and if there are any difficulties with "control" it is advisable to use one area consistently—for example, the thigh.

In diabetic emergencies soluble insulin is usually given intravenously, or occasionally intramuscularly (see page 26). Nasal insulin preparations are under investigation but not yet available.

Injection of insulin

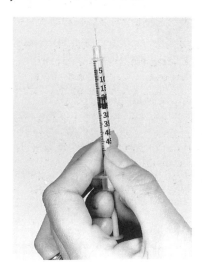

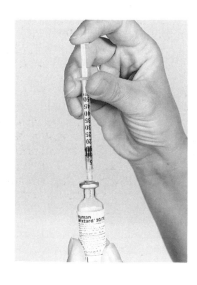

Drawing up the insulin

(1) Clean the top of the insulin bottle with industrial methylated spirit.

(2) Draw air into the syringe to the number of marks of insulin required and inject this into the insulin bottle; then draw the required dose of insulin into the syringe, and before withdrawing the needle from the insulin bottle, expel the air bubble if one has formed.

If clear and cloudy insulins are to be mixed, inject the correct number of marks of air first into the cloudy insulin bottle; withdraw the needle from the cloudy bottle; inject the air into the clear bottle, and withdraw the insulin into the syringe; finally, insert the needle into the cloudy bottle and withdraw the insulin.

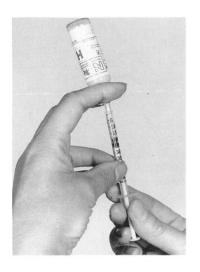

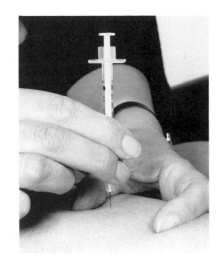

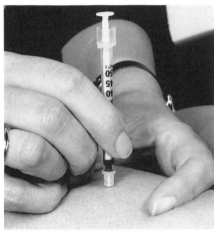

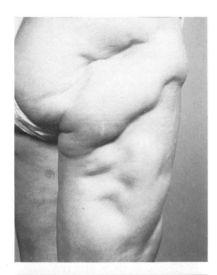

Injection technique

(1) The skin need not be specially cleaned; repeated application of spirit hardens the skin.

(2) Stretching the skin at the injection site is the best way to obtain a painless injection; in thin people it may be necessary to pinch the skin between thumb and forefinger of the left hand.

(3) The needle should be inserted briskly at almost 90° to the skin to almost its whole length (needles are usually 0·9 cm to 1·6 cm long).

(4) Inject the insulin by depressing the plunger. It is not necessary to pull back the plunger beforehand.

(5) Withdraw the needle and press briefly on the injection site with cotton wool.

(6) Replace the needle cover and return the whole syringe–needle unit to its container. Keep it in the refrigerator. Plastic syringes can be used for up to one month or until the scale becomes indistinct; disposable needles are used until they are blunt. Plastic syringes should not be kept in any form of preservative.

Problems associated with insulin injection

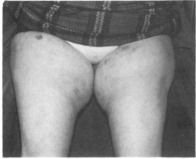

Many patients develop some blurring of vision soon after starting insulin, which makes reading difficult. This is due to a change of lens refraction and corrects itself within two to three weeks. Transient oedema of the feet is not uncommon during the first few weeks of insulin treatment.

Fat atrophy is rarely seen since the introduction of purified insulins. If it has occurred injection of insulin at the edge of the hollow towards the centre promotes filling out.

Fatty lumps at injection sites are common, and occasionally so large as to be unsightly. Their cause is not known but they sometimes develop if injections are repeatedly given over a very limited area of skin. For this reason it is best to vary the site from day to day. They are rarely troublesome, but once present they tend to persist.

Red itchy marks at injection sites after starting insulin are now rare and if they do occur usually disappear spontaneously. If they are troublesome adding hydrocortisone to the insulin bottle so that each dose contains about 1 mg eliminates the problem.

Insulin allergy causing urticaria is very rare indeed. If it occurs, desensitisation may be needed. Abscesses at injection sites are also remarkably rare.

Continuous subcutaneous insulin infusion

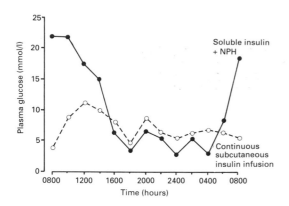

The technique of infusing insulin throughout 24 hours with pre-prandial boosts requires sophisticated and expensive infusion pumps, which are usually worn on a belt and attached to a subcutaneous cannula. Very tight diabetic control over long periods of time can be achieved by this technique if the user is prepared to take considerable trouble with its detailed application. Several problems have, however, been reported, notably rapid development of ketoacidosis if there is a technical pump failure or disconnection, infection, and sometimes considerable weight gain. The technique is also very expensive and costly to maintain. Modern insulin regimens, delivery devices, and insulin preparations can achieve a level of control often as good as continuous subcutaneous insulin infusion, which is now chiefly a research tool. Advice on this technique and the appropriate pumps is available only in a few specialised centres.

The illustration of porcine insulin crystals was reproduced, by permission, from *Insulin: Islet Pathology, Islet Function, Insulin Treatment*, ed Rolf Luft, published by Nordisk Insulinlaboratorium.

ASSESSMENT OF DIABETIC CONTROL: ADJUSTMENT OF INSULIN DOSE

Blood glucose measurement

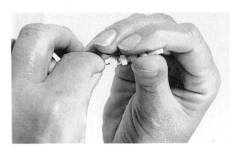

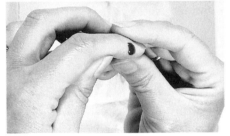

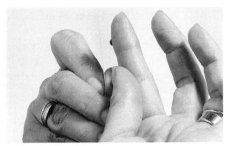

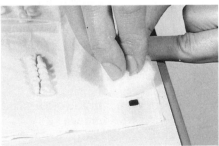

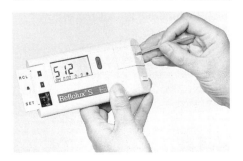

Blood glucose concentrations can be measured very simply by nurses at the bedside or by patients at home. Most diabetic patients, especially those taking insulin, find this technique extremely valuable. Patients should be taught very carefully to interpret the results. Not all patients can cope with the techniques required and it is not suitable for everyone: many older non-insulin dependent patients will find urine testing simple and adequate.

For many who decide to measure their own blood glucose concentrations it is sufficient to use blood glucose strips read by eye (see below), and expensive meters are unnecessary. Others obtain better results using a meter and gain considerable reassurance from the readings. A high degree of accuracy is not needed, but if the technique of performing the test is poor, results will be hopelessly inaccurate whichever method is used.

Technique

Obtaining the blood—The blood can be obtained by pricking a finger or, less easily, an earlobe (using a mirror). The best instrument to use is a purpose made needle (for example, Monolet (Sherwood) and Unilet G (Owen Mumford)). Several spring loaded prickers are available which simplify the task and ensure that an adequate drop of blood is obtained: they include the Autoclix (BM Diagnostics) and Glucolet (Bayer Diagnostics).

The test strip—The test strips are read by eye or by meter. The following strips are available: ExacTech (Medisense), BM-Test 1-44 (BM Diagnostics), Dextrostix (Bayer Diagnostics), Hypoguard GA (Hypoguard), and Glucostix (Bayer Diagnostics). It is very important to remember that blood glucose readings at the top of the scale of each of the strips represent minimum values and actual blood glucose concentrations could be much higher.

Blood glucose meters—Several meters are now available (the manufacturers' instructions should be followed very closely): ExacTech (MediSense); Reflolux (BM Diagnostics); Hypo-Count MXR, Hypo-Count MXA, and Hypo-Count GA (Hypoguard); and Glucometer (Bayer Diagnostics).

Capillary blood samples—If patients cannot cope with self-measurement of blood glucose but can manage to take capillary blood they can take their samples to hospital in simple plastic tubes coated with heparin and fluoride (Sarstedt tubes) and have their home blood glucose profiles measured at the diabetic clinic.

Purposes of home blood glucose measurements

The purposes of monitoring blood glucose are threefold: (*a*) as a spot check to detect hypoglycaemia; (*b*) to assess control in times of illness; (*c*) to assess the blood glucose profile over 24 hours.

Detecting hypoglycaemia

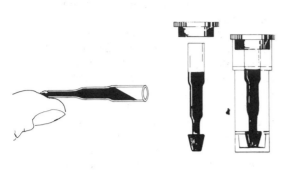

Sarstedt tubes for collecting capillary blood.

Detection of hypoglycaemia is one of the most important benefits of home measurement of glucose values. Thus the blood glucose concentration may be measured if the patient is uncertain about suspected hypoglycaemic symptoms, or if relatives suspect hypoglycaemia when a child behaves abnormally, becomes unconscious, or develops an epileptic convulsion. Home measurement is invaluable in preventing serious hypoglycaemia, since diabetic patients can discover for themselves the times of day when they are most susceptible to this hazard. In particular, measurement at bedtime in those prone to nocturnal hypoglycaemia is valuable: if the blood glucose is low (in general less than 5 mmol/l) extra carbohydrate may prevent hypoglycaemia. The same applies on other occasions when hypoglycaemia could be hazardous—for example, before driving long distances.

Blood glucose assessment during illness

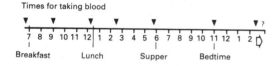

If blood glucose concentration is high during illness take extra insulin

The discovery of isolated high blood glucose readings in a symptomless diabetic patient is of limited value. During illness, however, when blood glucose concentrations tend to be high and accompanied by heavy glycosuria, raised blood glucose values may be a valuable guide to the need for extra insulin. If the level is above about 15 mmol/l an additional dose of a soluble insulin (about 8 units) would usually be quite safe. Random blood glucose readings may also help when particularly fine control is needed—for example, during pregnancy.

Blood glucose profiles

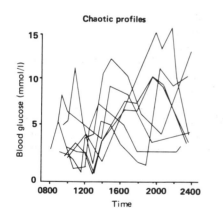

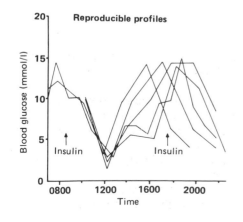

Assessment by insulin treated patients of the daily fluctuations of their blood glucose values results in a much greater understanding by patients and doctors of both diabetic control and the effects of different insulin preparations. Home blood glucose measurement is now an important educational exercise for seriously motivated and well organised diabetic patients. It is not suitable for all patients, and those who lack the necessary enthusiasm are better off using more traditional methods of urine testing: their blood glucose profiles may in any case be chaotic and differ from day to day and may thus be unhelpful in improving control.

Reproducible blood glucose profiles are valuable in making rational adjustments to treatment. They can show not only the times of the peaks and troughs of blood glucose concentration but also the duration of action of a given insulin preparation in an individual patient. Indeed, the effect of individual insulins varies considerably between patients, to the extent that a soluble insulin may have a more prolonged effect in one person than isophane in another.

Home blood glucose monitoring by the correct technique combined with the ability to understand the true significance of the readings, represents a very important advance in diabetic care. On the other hand obsessional patients who perform tests too often with frequent alterations of insulin dose, cause themselves protracted misery and often disabling hypoglycaemia. While this approach sometimes evolves as a result of the patient's personality, such techniques are all too often encouraged by medical attendants.

The aim is to maintain blood glucose in an acceptable range, usually about 4–10 mmol/l. Excursions outside this range are inevitable on occasions, leading either to transient hypoglycaemia or equally transient hyperglycaemia. Thus the occasional high blood glucose readings in an otherwise satisfactory profile can be ignored.

Good techniques for blood glucose assessment

- Perform just one blood glucose measurement daily (or occasionally on alternate days), except in times of illness, when more frequent testing is needed (see page 18)
- Timing (see chart)—Perform the daily blood glucose measurement at different times so that over several weeks an idea of the profile can be created (that is, the commonest times for high or low blood glucose readings—the peaks and troughs). For non-insulin dependent patients, especially those treated by diet alone, the fasting blood glucose concentration can provide a good guide to control. Otherwise patients can adopt the practice described above
- Aims—Patients need to understand that in insulin dependent diabetes blood glucose concentration fluctuates substantially. This does not indicate "brittle" diabetes (see page 21) and transient high blood glucose concentrations are not necessarily damaging to health

Guidelines to adjusting the insulin dose
- Changes in insulin dose should be made only once or twice weekly (except in times of illness, when more frequent changes may be needed)
- Insulin adjustment should be made according to peaks and troughs determined by the blood glucose profile: the adjustment should be to the dose preceding the peak or trough, not after the blood glucose reading has been taken (see diagram below)
- Changes in insulin dose at any one time should normally be kept within 10–20% of the existing daily dose—for example, a change of 4–8 units may be made in a patient taking a total daily dose of 40 units.

Patients should not respond to isolated high blood glucose readings by taking extra insulin: this causes a worsening of blood glucose oscillations rather than an improvement in their blood glucose profile.

Adjustments after assessment of blood glucose profiles

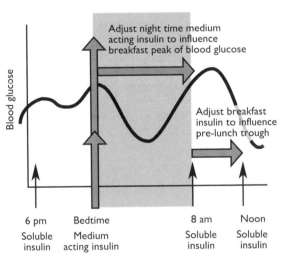

When consistent daily fluctuations of blood glucose have been shown, treatment should be modified, aiming chiefly to eliminate hypoglycaemic episodes and thereafter to obtain better control by increasing the blood glucose in the troughs and decreasing it at the peaks.

To *increase* blood glucose in the troughs:

(*a*) Eat more carbohydrate at or *before* the times when blood glucose values are at their lowest; the exact amount of extra carbohydrate can be determined only by trial and error.

(*b*) Reduce the dose of insulin *before* the trough.

To *decrease* blood glucose in the peaks:

(*a*) Reduce by a little the amount of carbohydrate taken at the meals which precede the peaks by two or three hours.

(*b*) Increase the dose of insulin before the peak.

Soluble insulin should be altered to change blood glucose concentration within six hours. Medium acting insulin should be altered to change blood glucose in six to 12 hours. The duration of insulin action varies considerably, however, and these figures provide only a rough guide.

Adjusting the insulin dose according to urine tests

Urine test				
	Breakfast	Lunch	Dinner	Bedtime
Weekly	✓	✓	✓	✓
Alternate days	✓			✓
Daily	✓ Day 1	✓ Day 2	✓ Day 3	✓ Day 4

For patients taking mixed insulins (with soluble and medium acting insulin each given twice daily)—If the urine test shows a large amount of glucose:

Before breakfast—increase the evening medium acting insulin.
Before lunch—increase the morning soluble insulin.
Before evening meal—increase the morning medium acting insulin.
Before bedtime—increase the evening soluble insulin.

For patients taking twice daily unmixed insulin injections—If the urine test shows a large amount of glucose:

Before lunch or evening meal—increase the morning dose.
Before bedtime or breakfast—increase the evening dose.

Haemoglobin A₁ (glycated haemoglobin)

1992	MAY	1992

SUN	MON	TUE	WED	THUR	FRI	SAT
					1	2
3	4				8	9
10	11	Haemoglobin A₁ in May			15	16
17	18				22	23
	25	26	27	28	29	30

1992	APRIL	1992

SUN	MON	TUE	WED	THUR	FRI	SAT
		1	2	3	4
5	6				10	11
12	13	Blood glucose in April			17	18
19	20				24	25
26	27	28	29	30		

Persistent hyperglycaemia modifies (glycates) haemoglobin A. Measurement of this haemoglobin fraction as a method of assessing diabetic control is unique in reflecting blood glucose concentrations in a period of about four weeks before the sample is taken. Unlike blood glucose concentrations, glycated haemoglobin concentrations do not fluctuate from hour to hour, so they are useful in the long term assessment of control and may identify patients whose control is not good but who prepare themselves for their clinic attendance. When pregnancies are planned, haemoglobin A₁ measurement may prove helpful in establishing optimum control before conception. It is frustrating to find that even in those whose control is thought to be satisfactory haemoglobin A₁ values are often raised; and sometimes a normal haemoglobin A₁ value is achieved only at the dangerous expense of nocturnal hypoglycaemia.

	Affinity chromatography (Abbott automated)	Immuno-assay	Ion exchange chromatography	Agar gel electrophoresis
Measures	"HbA₁ᴄ"	HbA₁ᴄ	HbA₁	HbA₁
Normal range	4·0–6·0%	4·0–6·0%	5·0–7·5%	5·0–7·5%
HbF	↔	↓	↑	↑
HbC, HbS	↔	↓	↓ or ↔	↓ or ↔
Lipaemia	↔	↔	↑	↔
Renal failure	↔	↔	↑	↔
Aspirin	↔	↔	↑	↑
Haemolysis Blood loss	↓	↓	↓	↓

There are now several methods for determining glycated haemoglobin: these determine either the fraction HbA_{1c} alone or total glycated haemoglobin (HbA_1), which represents the sum of subfractions HbA_{1a}, HbA_{1b}, and HbA_{1c}. Interference by abnormal haemoglobins, slow performance, and cost determine which method is selected for routine use. The four most commonly used techniques are listed in the table, together with their normal ranges and potential errors.

I thank Mrs V Brown for her help with the photographs.

Necrobiosis lipoidica diabeticorum

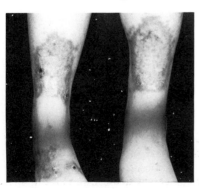

Necrobiosis is an uncommon and unsightly blemish of the skin which affects a few diabetic women. It is unrelated to microvascular complications. The shin is the most common site. The lesions show rather atrophic skin at the centre with obviously dilated capillaries (telangiectasis) and a slight raised pinkish rim; ulceration sometimes occurs. The lesions are indolent and rarely resolve. There is no effective treatment although steroid applications and even injection have been attempted.

THE UNSTABLE
INSULIN DEPENDENT PATIENT

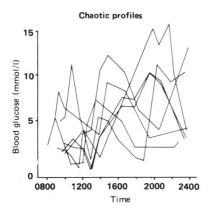

Chaotic profiles

- Identify technical errors
- Give the best diabetic regimen
- Search for other illness
- Seek social or psychological problems

Blood glucose concentrations inevitably oscillate considerably over 24 hours in most insulin treated diabetic patients. If these swings are used as a definition of instability then many patients might be classified as unstable. Indeed, the ardent desire of some doctors to "stabilise" diabetic patients sometimes leads patients to undertake innumerable blood and urine tests, to keep obsessional records, and to make themselves thoroughly miserable. The failure to succeed leads to recriminations, admissions to hospital, and absence from work. This form of physician induced unstable diabetes is made worse by the inappropriate use of home blood glucose monitoring. It needs considerable patience to unravel the effects of such advice, but a more relaxed approach together with fewer tests can have a remarkable effect.

Very unstable diabetes (sometimes described as "brittle") disrupts the lives of a small group of insulin treated diabetics with repeated admissions to hospital due to either hypoglycaemia or ketoacidosis. Home life, school, and work are totally disrupted. I doubt whether, with very few exceptions, this is a special type of diabetes: it most commonly occurs in teenage girls, it is almost always temporary, and the problems appear to vanish as life itself stabilises with employment or marriage.

Disruptive diabetes has several causes, ranging from simple technical errors to gross deceptions of great ingenuity. Management of these patients therefore demands time and patience: the doctor must identify any technical errors, recommend the best possible diabetic treatment, search for intercurrent illness, and seek social or psychological problems which might cause the patient to manipulate his or her diabetes.

Identifying technical problems

Check
- Injection technique
- Visual acuity
- Insulin strength and types
- Urine and blood glucose testing techniques

The technique of injecting insulin should be checked, injection sites inspected, and equipment scrutinised. Sometimes, especially in elderly patients, poor visual acuity makes drawing up of insulin extremely inaccurate. The insulin bottles themselves should also be checked for the type and strength of insulin. Techniques of urine and blood glucose testing must be observed and checked with laboratory results. Adequate understanding of diet should be verified.

The dose and type of insulin should be adjusted to the best possible regimen (ideal insulin regimens have been described elsewhere). A few unstable diabetic patients may benefit from continuous subcutaneous insulin infusion, which may also alleviate unpleasant hypoglycaemic episodes.

19

The unstable insulin dependent patient

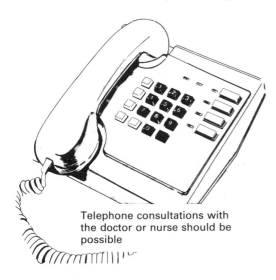

Telephone consultations with the doctor or nurse should be possible

If recurrent hypoglycaemic episodes are the chief problem then careful education is needed to eliminate them; careful attention needs to be given not only to the dose of insulin but also to timing and amount of food, the effects of exercise, and the judicious use of home measurement of blood glucose. Sometimes excessive amounts of insulin, especially soluble insulin, may cause severe hypoglycaemia. Improvement results from reducing the dose of insulin.

In a few women menstruation regularly causes severe upset of diabetes; control usually deteriorates in the premenstrual phase, causing ketoacidosis at times, followed by a decrease in insulin requirement and sometimes troublesome hypoglycaemia. A carefully planned campaign of insulin adjustment usually overcomes this problem.

Perhaps above all, these patients need encouragement and restoration of self-confidence together with the reassurance that they are neither physically nor mentally abnormal. The home telephone number of the doctor or the nurse offers added security. If at all possible unstable patients should not be admitted to hospital. If all these measures fail, however, and life is still disrupted by the diabetes, then admission is after all required.

Admission to hospital

At one clinic of yours which I attended, you asked me if I was taking overdoses. I was stupid and did not admit this until December 1981. I am still not as well balanced as I would like, but I am better than I was!

Letter from a patient.

In hospital the nursing staff take over the administration of insulin completely—both the procedure of drawing up the insulin and giving the injections. If some measure of stability is then achieved the patient's equipment is returned for self-injection: if chaos resumes it seems likely that the patient is either incompetent or cheating.

If diabetes continues to cause disruption even when the nursing staff are giving insulin injections some form of manipulation should be suspected. Some patients use great ingenuity: insulin may just be concealed in a locker, but it has also been found inside transistor radios, in the false bottoms of jewelry boxes, and taped outside hospital lavatory windows.

Manipulation should be suspected in patients whose lives are totally disrupted by their diabetes. A careful history may reveal slips which give the vital clue. For instance, one teenager developed profound hypoglycaemia two days after apparently "stopping insulin"; another, whose life was spent in and out of hospital with hypoglycaemia or ketoacidosis, claimed to be perfectly stable in betweeen, presenting a whole volume of negative urine tests. Even constant insulin infusion does not solve the problem, especially when the patient replaces the insulin in the syringe with water.

When there is strong evidence of manipulation, I usually hint at the possibility to the patient and his or her parents without accusation. The technique is sometimes successful and gratitude considerable.

Emotional, social, or psychiatric causes underlie disruptive diabetes and the desire to manipulate the situation to cause widespread havoc among families. Teenage defiance is a common cause. Quiet support of families at these difficult times helps to overcome what is almost always a temporary phase. Careful inquiry should establish whether or not there is a family strife. Psychiatric advice should not be sought unless there is evidence of true psychiatric disorder; otherwise, confrontation with a psychiatrist may provoke even more aggression. None the less, a few patients remain incapable of independent existence, and whether they are children or adults some form of institutional care has to be considered.

Various disorders, especially infections and some endocrine disorders, may alter the insulin requirements, although they rarely cause the type of instability already described.

Falsified urine chart from a very unstable teenage patient.

HYPOGLYCAEMIA

Hypoglycaemia is the major hazard of insulin treatment. Patients may experience the symptoms of hypoglycaemia when the blood concentration is less than 2·5 mmol/l but individual susceptibility varies considerably. The risks are small in most patients, but because they exist at all patients taking insulin are barred from certain occupations such as driving trains or buses. All patients taking insulin whose diabetes is reasonably well controlled will experience hypoglycaemia at some stage. At its mildest it is no more than a slight inconvenience, but at its severest, when unconsciousness can occur, it is both a hazard and an embarrassment. Hypoglycaemia occurs infrequently in patients taking oral hypoglycaemics.

All patients taking insulin must be carefully taught about the cause, symptoms, and treatment of hypoglycaemia.

KING'S COLLEGE HOSPITAL—DIABETIC DEPARTMENT

HYPOGLYCAEMIA ("hypo" "insulin reaction")

This is when the blood sugar goes too low in diabetics taking insulin.

Symptoms are sweating, shaking, tingling round the mouth, hazy eyesight or seeing double, slow thinking, in children naughtiness.

Causes are late meal, too little carbohydrate, extra exercise, too much insulin.

Cure is to take carbohydrate - preferably 3 dextrosol tablets, glucose, sugar (2 large lumps), barley sugar, Lucozade.

Symptoms will soon wear off.

If in doubt about an attack, take sugar.

Always carry some form of SUGAR with you

KCH 333

Symptoms

Early warning	Shaking, trembling
	Sweating
	Pins and needles in lips and tongue
	Hunger
	Palpitations
	Headache (occasionally)
Neuroglycopenia:	
Mild	Double vision
	Difficulty in concentrating
	Slurring of speech
More advanced	Confusion
	Change of behaviour
	Truculence
	Naughtiness in children
Unconsciousness	Restlessness with sweating
	Epileptic fits, especially in children
	Hemiplegia, especially in
	elderly people (but rare)

Most patients experience the early warning symptoms of hypoglycaemia and can take sugar before more serious symptoms develop. With increasing duration of diabetes in those who are very tightly controlled and in older patients there is a tendency for the early warning symptoms not to occur, and patients develop the more serious problems. Although this lack of warning has been attributed to autonomic neuropathy, I doubt whether this is generally the case, although β blockers occasionally have this effect. Friends and relations are then more often aware of hypoglycaemia than the patients themselves, observing them to be slow witted with a vacant expression and perspiring face and hands: they should give the patient sugar immediately.

Patients who become unconscious from hypoglycaemia should be taken to hospital immediately. Brain damage and death do not usually occur because the blood glucose concentration tends to increase spontaneously as the effect of the insulin wears off. Many diabetics, especially children, need reassurance that they will not die in their sleep. Nevertheless, a very small number of otherwise unexplained deaths at night have been reported in young insulin dependent diabetic patients and may have been caused by hypoglycaemia. Deaths from prolonged hypoglycaemia are most likely to occur after insulin overdoses, as a result of either a suicide or murder attempt, but even in these circumstances most patients recover.

Causes of hypoglycaemia

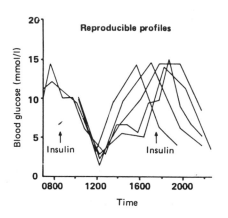

In every patient taking insulin the blood glucose concentration shows peaks and troughs, which can be most clearly shown by home measurement of blood glucose. Since the lowest blood glucose concentrations, when the symptoms of hypoglycaemia are most likely to appear, occur at different times in each patient, it is a great advantage if individual patients know when their own troughs are likely to occur. The commonest times are before lunch and during the night.

Apart from the natural troughs in blood glucose concentrations, other events likely to provoke hypoglycaemic attacks are: insufficient carbohydrate in meals; delayed meals; physical activity; and errors of insulin dosage. Really severe physical activity, such as swimming very long distances, is a powerful stimulus of hypoglycaemia, and as much as 40–50 g additional carbohydrate may be needed to prevent it.

Hypoglycaemia is particularly likely to occur shortly after stabilisation of new patients, as their insulin requirements may decline considerably; the insulin dose should therefore always be reduced before they leave hospital.

Some patients have reported an exacerbation of loss of warning of hypoglycaemia during treatment with human insulin. It is not known why this might occur, but these patients should be transferred back to porcine preparations of insulin.

Hypoglycaemia is also troublesome when insulin requirements insidiously decrease at the onset of certain disorders, including Addison's disease, hypopituitarism, and malabsorption syndromes.

Treatment

Items containing 10 g of carbohydrate

Milk ....200 ml ($\frac{1}{3}$ pint)

Lucozade ....60 ml (4 tablespoons)

Ribena ....15 ml (1 tablespoon)

Coca Cola ....90 ml

Sugar ....2 teaspoons

Sugar lumps (small) 3

Dextrosol tablets 3

Glucagon kit

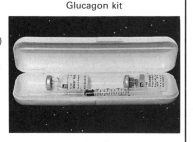

Dr Charles Fletcher's account of hypoglycaemia

My main problem has always been hypoglycaemia. At first I was nearly always aware of it by day and woke at night, because of the adrenaline response. But, particularly in the past 20 years, it gradually became more difficult. I may now feel normal and do ordinary tasks quite easily with blood sugar as low as 2·5 mmol/l (45 mg/100 ml). Sometimes diplopia, dysphasia, weariness, or inability to think may lead me to do a blood sugar. But I often become too muddled to know what is wrong, and I have had to thank my wife, my children, and many generations of housemen, registrars, and secretaries for spotting these low levels on many occasions. Before I retired 50% glucose was always available with syringe in a drawer in my desk. I became quite used to a quiet registrar's voice in outpatients (and elsewhere) saying, "I think, sir, a little extravenous glucose might help." Lucozade has been invaluable. I always have it available in th car, in the office, and at home. It is acceptably free from sugariness, it saves me chewing and choking on dry glucose tablets, and it is rapidly absorbed. My wife finds it much easier to get me to drink this than to take any other form of sugar when I am severely hypoglycaemic and refuse to acknowledge it. I have made it a rule, which I now keep, even when semi-comatose, that if my wife—or anyone else—tells me to take sugar I do so however sure I may be that I'm not hypoglycaemic. They have only been wrong on rare occasions. I am very sensitive to exercise, but for some reason I find it difficult always to suck prophylactic sweets on country walks or when digging or mowing in the garden.

BMJ 1980;**280**:1115–16.

Prevention is most important. *All diabetic patients should carry on their person and in their cars either sugar lumps, sweets, or dextrosol tablets (or sugar gel which may be squeezed around the gums).* They should take ample carbohydrate at the times when their blood glucose troughs occur and extra carbohydrate before vigorous exercise such as football.

If the early warning symptoms occur (table) they should take 10–20 g of sugar immediately. If the response is poor more can be taken. Unconscious patients should be given intravenous glucose (20–50 ml of 50% glucose) in hospital after blood has been taken for confirmatory analysis later. At home they can be given an injection of glucagon (1 mg intramuscularly), which quickly raises the blood glucose. It may be helpful and a great comfort to the relations of patients who are liable to become unconscious from hypoglycaemia to keep glucagon in a convenient place.

Patients who remain unconscious after prolonged hypoglycaemia are sometimes given treatment for cerebral oedema with intravenous mannitol and dexamethasone. They usually recover. It is very important to be certain of the correct diagnosis of unconsciousness.

Where human insulin is thought by patients to have exacerbated hypoglycaemia conversion back to porcine insulin is advised.

Hypoglycaemia due to oral hypoglycaemics is treated in the same way as described above, but patients usually require admission to hospital for continuous glucose infusion to avoid relapse to hypoglycaemia, which often occurs until the drug has been cleared from the circulation.

Management of patients with recurrent disabling hypoglycaemic episodes is described in the previous chapter.

DIABETIC EMERGENCIES

Ketoacidosis

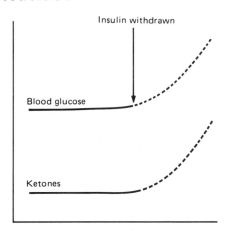

Ketoacidosis results from a lack of insulin. In practice it is usually due to:

(*a*) stopping insulin or reducing the dose—in error or deliberately;
(*b*) resistance to insulin during infections;
(*c*) the unrecognised onset of insulin dependent diabetes.

The clinical onset of ketoacidosis occurs over hours or days. Symptoms of uncontrolled diabetes are always present. Vomiting in an insulin dependent patient is always serious. Patients usually consult their doctors during the preceding days, but the presence of uncontrolled diabetes is nearly always overlooked. Diabetic control should always be assessed if a diabetic patient becomes unwell for any reason. Almost all cases of ketoacidosis can be prevented.

Preventing ketoacidosis

> **Insulin should never be stopped**

> KING'S COLLEGE HOSPITAL—DIABETIC DEPARTMENT
>
> **ILLNESS AND INFECTION**
>
> During illness or infection your blood sugar level **may** rise, causing you to feel dry, thirsty and pass too much urine. Urine tests may become sugary (2%) every time.
>
> You **MUST** continue to take your normal insulin dose. **NEVER** stop it. You may need an increased dose if your urine tests are bad. If you are vomiting, consult your Doctor or the Diabetic Clinic at once. If you are unable to eat, take your carbohydrate portions in liquid form—e.g. milk, Lucozade, Ribena.
>
> Test your urine twice a day or even more frequently.
>
> If you continue to feel unwell, consult your Doctor.

During any illness or infection the blood glucose concentration tends to increase and diabetic control deteriorates. Most patients then need a larger dose of insulin than usual, and some who normally take tablets may need insulin just during the illness. The increased need for insulin occurs even when appetite declines or vomiting begins.

It is helpful to give every insulin dependent patient a small printed card with the simple instruction "Insulin should never be stopped." Stopping or even reducing insulin during the course of an illness often leads to diabetic ketoacidosis.

When a diabetic person is ill the normal insulin dose should be continued, carbohydrate taken in some palatable fluid form, and the urine tested regularly—four times a day if necessary. Blood glucose should also be tested. If heavy glycosuria (2%) persists or blood glucose readings greater than 15 mmol/l are obtained the dose of short acting (soluble) insulin should be increased. Additional doses of soluble insulin (about 8 units) may also be given at noon or bedtime when control is very poor. If vomiting continues without remission for more than a few hours admission to hospital for treatment with intraveneous fluids and insulin is advisable to prevent ketoacidosis.

Recognising ketoacidosis

> **Symptoms of ketoacidosis**
>
> ● Drowsiness
> ● Dehydration
> ● Overbreathing
> ● Acetone on breath
> ● Hypotension
> ● Gastric splash

Dehydration is the most obvious clinical feature of patients with ketoacidosis. They are also drowsy, but rarely unconscious—"diabetic coma" is an inappropriate description; they are overbreathing, but not usually breathless; their breath smells of acetone (though many people cannot smell this); and many also have a gastric splash. More severe cases are hypothermic and hypotensive. Aketotic cases are similar but without overbreathing or the smell of acetone.

Diagnosis

- Blood glucose
- Serum potassium and sodium
- Acid-base status
- Urea, creatinine
- Plasma ketones (Ketostix)
- Blood count
- Blood culture (when indicated)

The diagnosis of ketoacidosis is confirmed by laboratory tests.

Urine test shows heavy glycosuria and ketonuria.

Blood glucose concentrations may range from slightly increased to extreme hyperglycaemia. The blood glucose concentration itself does not usually indicate the severity of the illness.

Blood acid-base state—pH ranges from normal to 6·9. The bicarbonate value is depressed.

Plasma ketones are easily detectable with Ketostix. In patients with ketoacidosis the results on plasma Ketostix testing should be + + or + + +. The plasma Ketostix test is useful if acidosis is thought to be due to another cause, such as lactic acidosis.

Electrolytes—The serum potassium concentration is usually but not always raised. This measurement is vital, and lifesaving treatment is needed to maintain potassium values in the normal range. The sodium concentration is normal or reduced and urea and creatinine concentrations are often raised through dehydration.

Blood count—If a blood count is performed the white cell count is often spuriously raised to $15-20 \times 10^9/l$ even in the absence of infection.

Treatment

Physiological saline:*	1 l in first half hour	$-\frac{1}{2}$ h
	1 l over next hour	$\frac{1}{2} - 1\frac{1}{2}$ h
	1 l over next hour	$1\frac{1}{2} - 2\frac{1}{2}$ h
	1 l over next 2 hours	$2\frac{1}{2} - 4\frac{1}{2}$ h
	1 l over next 3 hours	$4\frac{1}{2} - 7\frac{1}{2}$ h
	1 l over next 4 hours	$7\frac{1}{2} - 11\frac{1}{2}$ h
Total:	6 l	$11\frac{1}{2}$ hours

*Change to dextrose 10% when blood glucose is less than 10 mmol/l.

(1) Insert a nasogastric tube (unless the patient is fully conscious). Do not allow any fluids by mouth; if patients are thirsty they may suck ice.

(2) Give intravenous fluids. The regimen needs to be modified according to age, weight, and the presence of cardiac disease. In seriously ill patients or those with cardiac disease a catheter for measuring central venous pressure is useful. A suitable regimen for most patients is shown. Saline 0·9% is used.

The fluid should be changed to dextrose 10% once the blood glucose concentration has fallen to less than 10 mmol/l. The rate of infusion is determined by individual need but at this stage should probably be about 1 litre every 8 hours.

(3) Start intravenous (or intramuscular) soluble insulin immediately.

Insulin treatment

Intravenous insulin—Soluble insulin is diluted in 0·9% saline in a syringe, at a concentration of 1 U/ml. It is given by infusion pump (or paediatric drip set) at 6 U/h (0·1 U/kg/h for children) until the blood glucose concentration is less than 10 mmol/l. Blood glucose should fall at a rate of about 5 mmol/l/h. Then the dose may be reduced to 3 U/h. Higher infusion rates are rarely needed; when they are needed in insulin resistant cases the rate should be doubled or quadrupled, etc. The insulin infusion is continued until the patient is well enough to eat. Preprandial subcutaneous soluble insulin is then given and intravenous insulin discontinued after the meal. Intravenous insulin should not be stopped before subcutaneous insulin has been given.

Intramuscular insulin—Soluble insulin 20 units is given as a loading dose, then 6 units every hour until blood glucose is less than 10 mmol/l, then continued at 2 hourly intervals. As with intravenous insulin, higher doses are rarely needed.

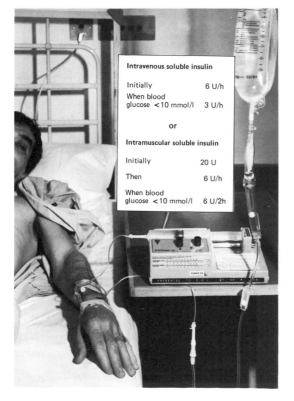

Intravenous soluble insulin	
Initially	6 U/h
When blood glucose <10 mmol/l	3 U/h
or	
Intramuscular soluble insulin	
Initially	20 U
Then	6 U/h
When blood glucose <10 mmol/l	6 U/2h

Potassium chloride administration

Serum value (mmol/l)	<3.5	3.5–4	4–5	>5
Administer	40 mmol/l	30 mmol/l	20 mmol/l	0

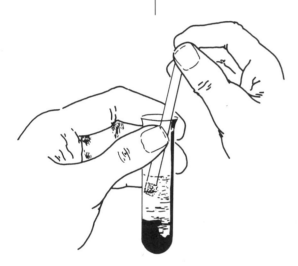

Plasma Ketostix test

0	+	++	+++
Not ketoacidosis		Ketoacidosis	

Potassium and sodium bicarbonate

Potassium chloride administration should usually start at about the second hour, preferably not before the serum potassium concentration is known. It should be withheld in exceptional cases of oliguria or anuria, or if the serum potassium value remains above 5 mmol/l. After the second hour, or earlier if the initial serum potassium value is normal or less than 4 mmol/l, 20 mmol of potassium chloride should be added to each litre of saline. If the serum potassium value falls below 3·5 mmol/l, 40 mmol should be used in each litre. The exact amount should be determined by serial serum potassium measurements—every two hours at first, then every four—and serum potassium maintained between 4 and 5 mmol/l. An electrocardiographic monitor should be set up; there is, however, no substitute for serial potassium measurements.

Sodium bicarbonate is not normally beneficial and is not given unless the blood pH value is less than 7·0 or the patient is shocked. If it is needed, aliquots of sodium bicarbonate (200 ml of 2·74% containing 65 mmol) with added potassium chloride (15 mmol) should be given over 30 to 60 minutes. This can be repeated if there is no response within one hour and if the patient's condition remains serious.

Treatment of the underlying condition—Underlying disease should be sought, especially respiratory or urinary infections, which may not be obvious at the beginning. Blood culture, culture of a mid-stream specimen of urine, and chest radiography are performed. There is no need to give antibiotics routinely. It is not usually difficult to distinguish a genuine surgical acute abdomen from the moderate pain and tenderness that are simply due to ketoacidosis.

Aketotic, hyperosmolar states—Management is exactly the same as that for ketoacidosis, except that 0·45% saline is given (if the serum sodium value is greater than 150 mmol/l), and a lower rate of insulin infusion (3 U/h) is often sufficient. In shocked and dehydrated patients prophylactic low dose subcutaneous heparin is considered. Patients who develop this condition are often elderly or West Indian, and they often turn out to be non-insulin dependent.

Lactic acidosis—These patients are profoundly ill and the cause of the acidosis must be sought and rigorously treated. They are often very insulin resistant and need large amounts of sodium bicarbonate. A plasma Ketostix value less than + + excludes ketoacidosis as a likely cause of the metabolic acidosis.

Management of diabetes during surgery

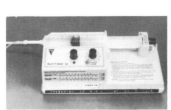
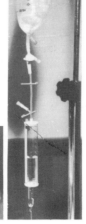

Continue insulin throughout
Intravenous insulin is best, either by drip or pump

The chief principle of diabetic management through any crisis in which patients cannot eat or drink for any reason is to *continue insulin administration*. The best method is to give the insulin by continuous intravenous infusion, either by infusion pump, directly from the drip bag, or using a paediatric drip set.

During surgery, management of the diabetic patient will depend on whether or not he or she needs insulin.

Surgery in insulin treated patients

Dextrose drip and variable rate insulin infusion

(1) Give normal insulin on the night before the operation.

(2) Early on the day of operation start an infusion of dextrose 10%, add 10 mmol KCl to each litre, and run at a *constant* rate appropriate to the patient's fluid requirements, usually 125 ml/h.

(3) Make up a solution of soluble insulin 1 U/ml saline in a syringe and infuse intravenously by a line piggybacked to the intravenous drip by using a syringe pump. The infusion rate should normally be as shown in regimen 1, but in resistant cases use regimen 2 or 3.

Blood glucose	Soluble insulin infusion rate		
	Regimen1	Regimen 2	Regimen 3
<4 mmol/l	0·5 U/h	1 U/h	2 U/h
4–15 mmol/l	2 U/h	4 U/h	8 U/h
>15 mmol/l	4 U/h	8 U/h	16 U/h
>20 mmol/l		Review	

Blood glucose is measured preoperatively and then 2 hourly until stable, then 6 hourly.

Urine tests should also be performed as a safeguard against erroneous ward blood glucose readings.

Regimen 1 is satisfactory for most cases; very severely ill patients, shocked patients, and those receiving steroids, salbutamol, or dopexamine infusions may need higher dose infusions, such as regimens 2 or 3, or occasionally even more.

Do not stop the insulin infusion since intravenous insulin lasts for only a few minutes.

Only if the patient becomes frankly hypoglycaemic (blood glucose <2 mmol/l) should insulin be stopped for up to 30 minutes.

For operations in which a patient is likely to be maintained on a drip for more than 12 hours a regimen is needed which can be continued for an indefinite period. Again there are two methods of administering the insulin: a variable rate infusion using a pump, or, if this is not available, a glucose-insulin infusion.

Note
- The rate of intravenous infusion must depend on the clinical state of the patient with regard to the volume depletion, cardiac failure, age, etc
- If the blood glucose is persistently >10 mmol/l the infusion should be changed to saline 0·9%
- Regular (at least daily) electrolyte measurements are required.

Glucose-insulin infusion (when no pump is available)

(1) Give normal insulin on the night before the operation.

(2) Begin an infusion of dextrose 10% containing 10 mmol KCl and soluble insulin 16 units per litre. Run it at a rate appropriate to the patient's fluid requirements, usually 125 ml/h. Adjust insulin dose as follows:

Blood glucose	Soluble insulin infusion
<4 mmol/l	8 U soluble insulin/l
4–15 mmol/l	16 U soluble insulin/l
>15 mmol/l	32 U soluble insulin/l
>20 mmol/l	Review

Blood glucose is measured 2 hourly until stable, then 6 hourly.

Urine tests should also be performed as a safeguard against erroneous ward blood glucose readings.

After recovery: changing to subcutaneous insulin

Use soluble insulin subcutaneously twice daily

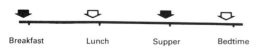

Optional extra doses at noon and midnight if blood glucose >15 mmol/l

Once the patient starts to eat and drink conversion back to subcutaneous insulin injections is undertaken as follows:
- Always change to subcutaneous insulin before breakfast and never in the evening
- Stop the insulin pump 30 minutes after the first subcutaneous insulin injection
- Insulin regimen and dose:

If the previous regimen is known then this should be given; if the patient is still in bed or unwell the total dose may need to be 10–20% more than usual

If the patient was not previously taking insulin predicting the requirement is not easy and the amount needs adjustment from day to day. Initially try soluble insulin 30–40 units daily in divided doses given four times daily.

Patients with hyperglycaemia often relapse after conversion back to subcutaneous insulin. When this happens there are three possible approaches: (1) Give additional doses of soluble insulin at any of the four injection times (before meals or bedtime). (2) Add intravenous insulin infusion temporarily while continuing the subcutaneous regimen until the blood glucose concentration is satisfactory. (3) Revert completely to the intravenous regimen, especially if the patient is unwell.

Surgery in non-insulin dependent patients

> - Omit usual treatment
> - Use insulin if diabetic control deteriorates
> - Maintain urine as well as blood glucose chart

Management of diabetic patients treated with diet or oral hypoglycaemic agents is more straightforward, so long as the diabetes is well controlled.

If the patient has well controlled diabetes (random blood glucose value < 12 mmol/l):

(1) Omit the tablet on the day of operation.

(2) Check the blood glucose concentration before and soon after operation; if the blood glucose value is over 12 to 15 mmol/l start soluble insulin.

If the diabetes is poorly controlled (random blood glucose > 15 mmol/l) the patient should be started on insulin before the operation, using one of the regimens described above.

DIABETIC COMPLICATIONS: RETINOPATHY

Microangiopathy:
Retinopathy
Nephropathy

Neuropathy

Macroangiopathy:
Atheroma
Medial calcification

Patients with longstanding diabetes may develop complications affecting the eyes or kidneys (microvascular complications), nerves, or major arteries.

The major arteries are affected by diabetes in two ways. Coronary artery disease is commoner in diabetic people than in non-diabetic people.

The greatest risk of large vessel disease occurs in those diabetic patients who develop proteinuria or microalbuminuria, suggesting widespread vascular damage. The distribution of arterial narrowing tends to be more distal than in non-diabetic people, whether in the coronary arteries or in the peripheral arteries affecting feet and legs. Medial arterial calcification (Monckeberg's sclerosis) is also substantially increased in patients with neuropathy and those with nephropathy. The functional effects of vascular calcification are uncertain.

Pattern of microvascular complications

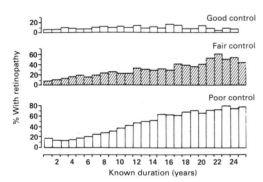

Adapted from Pirart J. *Diabete et Metabolisme* 1977; **3**: 97–107; fig 10.

The cause of the microvascular complications is not understood, but the most important influence is probably the quality of diabetic control over many years. There may also be a genetic influence, which can be detected in identical twins. Fortunately not all diabetic patients develop these complications, and probably as many as a fifth are spared altogether even after 40 or 50 years of diabetes.

Curiously, both retinopathy and neuropathy may occur in isolation, but serious nephropathy is always accompanied by retinopathy and usually by neuropathy as well.

Retinopathy

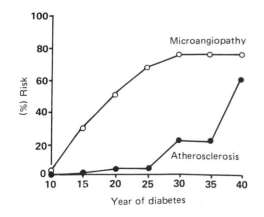

After 30 years of diabetes over 80% of patients will have retinopathy. In many cases this is a mild background retinopathy which changes little over the years. Rather unpredictably, however, changes may develop which threaten vision, generally from macular disease or vitreous haemorrhage. Since treatment is now available which can prevent blindness, it is essential to identify the lesions which are amenable to treatment before vision deteriorates.

Classification of retinopathy

Background retinopathy
Microaneurysms appear as tiny red dots and represent small capillary aneurysms or bulges. They are abnormally permeable but by themselves not harmful.

Diabetic complications: retinopathy

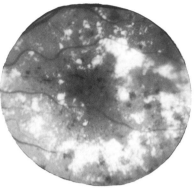
Background retinopathy: exudates encroaching on macula.

Severe exudative retinopathy.

Haemorrhages appear as small (dot) and large (blot) red spots on the retina. They are harmless unless they occur on the macula itself, when they can severely impair vision.

"Hard" exudates—These are yellow-white discrete patches which often occur in rings around leaking capillaries. They may coalesce to form extensive sheets of exudate. They cause blindness only when they occur in the macula.

Maculopathy—If hard exudates advance on to the macula, vision gradually declines and blindness eventually develops. Macular oedema also causes blindness: it may develop quite rapidly. Its recognition is difficult, but its presence is suggested by a grey discoloration at the macula.

Preproliferative lesions

Ischaemia of the retina probably predisposes to the development of dangerous formation of new vessels. An ophthalmologist should be consulted at this stage. The lesions are: (*a*) multiple cotton wool spots, which are indistinct and relatively large pale lesions, representing areas of capillary closure; (*b*) multiple large blot haemorrhages; (*c*) venous beading, loops, and reduplication; (*d*) arterial sheathing; and (*e*) atrophic looking retina.

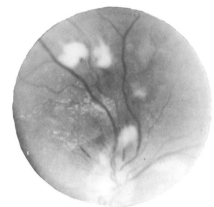
Cotton wool spots.

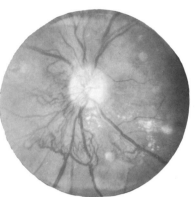
Disc new vessels.

Proliferative retinopathy

If there are peripheral new vessels the risk of serious vitreous haemorrhage is small, but new vessels on the disc are likely to develop. New vessels on the disc commonly bleed, causing preretinal haemorrhages and blindness from vitreous haemorrhage.

Advanced diabetic eye disease

The signs of advanced diabetic eye disease are: vitreous haemorrhage; fibrous tissue, which may shrink and cause retinal detachment; and rubeosis iridis and glaucoma—new vessels spread to the anterior chamber and affect the iris (rubeosis iridis). If the new vessels obstruct the outflow from the anterior chamber a most painful form of glaucoma occurs, sometimes requiring enucleation.

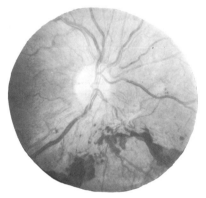
Preretinal haemorrhages.

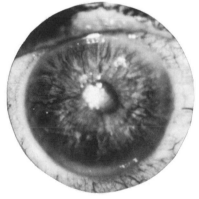
Rubeosis iridis.

Causes of blindness in diabetic patients

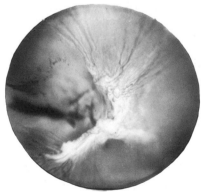
Advanced eye disease with fibrosis.

After 30 years of diabetes, about 7% of patients are blind: there are in all about 8000 registered blind diabetic people in England and Wales, most being over 60 years old.

Vitreous haemorrhage from new vessels occurs suddenly, painlessly, and without warning, and blindness rapidly develops. Some clearing of the haemorrhage is likely over the following weeks but recovery of vision becomes progressively less likely after repeated haemorrhage.

Maculopathy—Exudates or oedema that directly affect the macula cause blindness. The onset is gradual over weeks or months, during which vision gradually deteriorates.

Glaucoma and retinal detachment are other cause of blindness in diabetic retinopathy.

The lens—Lens opacities or cataracts develop more often in diabetic people than in non-diabetic people. There is a very rare form of rapidly developing cataract which occurs in some young patients.

29

Prevention of blindness

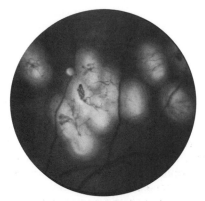

After a few days

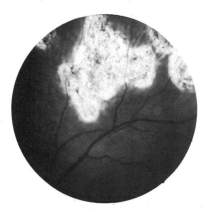

After a few months

Photocoagulation scars.

Retinopathy needs to be actively sought by physicians because if it is detected early enough blindness can be prevented by light coagulation with xenon arc or argon laser. The indications for photocoagulation are: (*a*) the presence of new vessels on the disc. Sometimes new vessels peripheral to the disc are treated as well, especially if they become preretinal, because they often herald the development of vessels on the disc; (*b*) the development of maculopathy either by exudates or oedema: this should be treated when visual acuity *begins* to decline—that is, a decrease of one or two lines on the Snellen chart. Once visual acuity is less than 6/36 the treatment is of no value.

Surgical treatment of blindness, including vitrectomy, will not be discussed here.

Clinical examination of the eyes and screening

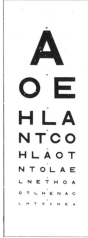

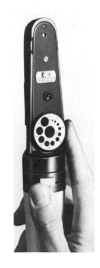

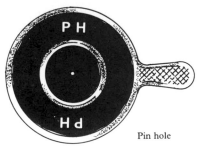

Pin hole

Visual acuity should be checked regularly, usually annually, but more often if required when retinopathy is present. Refraction should be performed with the patient wearing glasses or, if glasses are not available, by viewing the test chart through a "pin hole."

Retinal examination—Routine examination of the fundi should be performed on all diabetic patients: the pupils should be dilated and examined, preferably in a darkened room. Pupils should not be dilated if there is any suspicion of glaucoma. Tropicamide (Mydriacil) eye drops are recommended because the pupils recover from their action in two or three hours without the need for reversal with pilocarpine eye drops.

The fundi of all new patients should be examined. Ideally, visual acuity should be tested and a retinal examination performed each year. Examinations may be performed less often in short term symptomless patients without known retinopathy. Once retinopathy is present examinations should be performed every 6 to 12 months or more often if indicated. If the dates and results of eye examinations appear in a prominent place in the records, it becomes a simple matter to decide on the date of follow up examinations.

Indications for referral to an ophthalmologist

- Declining visual acuity from any cause
- Presence of proliferative or preproliferative changes
- Presence of exudates encroaching on the macula

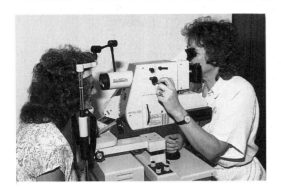

Screening methods

Conventional examination, using an ophthalmoscope in a darkened room with the pupil dilated. The observer, who should be suitably trained, can be a hospital doctor, general practitioner, or optometrist.

Retinal photography thorugh dilated pupils. Photographs may be taken either on polaroid film, providing a visible record in the patient's notes, or on 35 mm film, which is both cheaper and provides films of better quality. Films should be read by a trained observer.

When retinopathy is discovered patients should normally be referred for review to the local diabetic clinic unless there are the specific indications for a review by an ophthalmologist (see box).

The blind diabetic patient

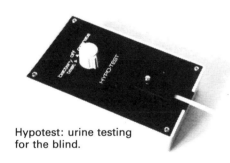

Hypotest: urine testing for the blind.

Once blind, the patient should register with the local authority because some amenities and a little financial help are available. Rehabilitation is available for suitable patients at the Royal National Institute for the Blind centre at Torquay, and some blind diabetic people are helped by guide dogs. Printing in Braille is valuable but many diabetic people cannot read it because of the impairment of fine sensation in their fingers. For insulin injections a preset syringe is available, but even more valuable is one of the insulin "pens" (Hypoguard Ltd, Ispwich, Suffolk), in which each palpable click corresponds to a single mark on the syringe. Urine tests can be performed using Diastix together with a Hypotest instrument, which gives an audible signal corresponding to the amount of glycosuria.

I thank Mr E W G Davies and Mr C Clements for their help in obtaining photographs of diabetic retinopathy. The photographs of the preset and Hypotest meter are reproduced by permission of Hypoguard Ltd. The third illustration is reproduced, with permission, from *Kidney International* 1974; **6**: 55.

DIABETIC NEUROPATHY—I: THE DIABETIC FOOT

Diabetic neuropathies constitute a diverse group of conditions. The commonest is a diffuse polyneuropathy which damages distal peripheral nerves (affecting chiefly the feet), together with the autonomic nervous system. It is a classic diabetic complication, gradually progressing (albeit at very variable rates) as the duration of diabetes lengthens and often, but not always, associated with other long term diabetic complications. In contrast mononeuropathies and acute painful neuropathies run a well defined cause from a relatively acute onset to a more or less complete recovery in 6 to 18 months. These reversible neuropathies, which may be the reason for initial presentation, occur at any stage of diabetes, are commoner in non-insulin dependent men, and are not necessarily associated with other diabetic complications.

Pressure neuropathies are commoner in diabetic people than in other people and include carpal tunnel syndrome (median nerve), ulnar neuropathy, and, rarely, foot drop (lateral popliteal nerve).

This chapter deals with peripheral neuropathy, in particular the diabetic foot; the next chapter deals with autonomic neuropathy; and the next mononeuropathies and acute painful neuropathies.

Symmetrical sensory neuropathy

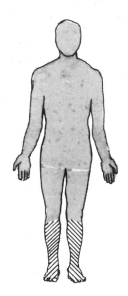

Diffuse neuropathy affects peripheral nerves symmetrically, chiefly those of the feet and legs. It is almost always sensory, though motor involvement causing weakness and wasting does occur rarely. Peripheral neuropathy is common in longstanding diabetic patients, but in older patients it may already be present at the onset of the diabetes. Progression of neuropathy may be reduced by good control of diabetes over many years; other agents which might help in this regard are gamolenic acid (evening primrose oil) and aldose reductase inhibitors, though more long term preventive studies are needed to establish their clinical role. Gangliosides do not have a convincing effect.

Neuropathy is usually symptomless and is therefore a hazard to the unwary patient. In more advanced neuropathies the patient is aware of sensory loss: numbness (and in some a sensation of coldness) may progressively worsen until there is almost complete anaesthesia below the knee, but this is not common. Reduced sensation in the feet may result in unnoticed trauma from ill fitting shoes, nails, or stones, walking barefoot, or burns from hot water bottles or sitting too close to a fire. Self inflicted wounds from crude attempts at chiropody are dangerous because they often become infected.

The diabetic foot

The three main factors that lead to tissue necrosis in the diabetic foot are neuropathy, infection, and ischaemia. Diabetic foot problems can be divided into those in which neuropathy predominate (neuropathic foot) and those where atherosclerosis is the main factor, though neuropathy may also be present to a variable degree (neuroischaemic foot). The features and complications of both these types of feet are listed in the box.

The Neuropathic ulcer

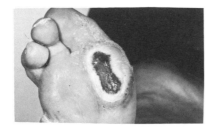

Ulcers develop at the tips of the toes and on the plantar surfaces of the metatarsal heads and are often preceded by callus formation. If the callus is not removed then haemorrhage and tissue necrosis occurs below the plaque of callus, which leads to ulceration. Ulcers can be secondarily infected by staphylococci, streptococci, coliforms, and anaerobic bacteria, which can quickly lead to cellulitis, abscess formation, and osteomyelitis. Sepsis complicating apical toe ulcers can lead to in situ thrombosis of the digital arteries, resulting in gangrene of the toe.

Treatment

Management of the ulcer falls into three parts: removal of callus, eradication of infection, and reduction of weight bearing forces.

Excess keratin should be pared away with a scalpel blade by the chiropodist to expose the floor of the ulcer and allow efficient drainage of the lesion. If the ulcer penetrates to bone a radiograph should be taken to assess the possibility of osteomyelitis.

A bacterial swab should be taken from the floor of the ulcer after the callus has been removed. A superficial ulcer may be treated on an outpatient basis and oral antibiotics prescribed according to the organisms isolated until the ulcer has healed. The most likely organisms to infect a superficial ulcer are staphylococci or streptococci. Thus treatment is started initially with penicillin V 500 mg four times a day and flucloxacillin 500 mg four times a day and adjusted when bacteriological culture results are available. The patient should be instructed to carry out daily dressing of the ulcer. A simple non-adherent dressing should be applied after cleaning the ulcer with physiological saline.

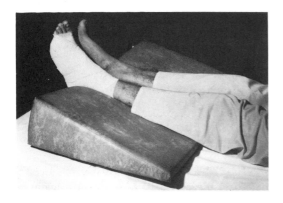

If the ulcer is associated with cellulitis, abscess, discoloration of surrounding skin, or crepitus (gas in soft tissues) the limb is threatened and urgent hospital admission should be arranged and the following regimen adopted:

(1) Bedrest.

(2) Intravenous antibiotics. In the first 24 hours before bacteriological cultures are available it is necessary to provide a wide spectrum of antibiotic cover. Thus quadruple therapy may be necessary consisting of amoxycillin 500 mg three times a day to treat streptococci, flucloxacillin 500 mg four times a day to treat staphylococci, metronidazole 400 mg three times a day to treat anaerobes and either ceftazidime 1 g three times a day or gentamicin 80 mg three times a day, depending on renal function, to treat Gram negative organisms. This treatment can be adapted when results of bacteriological culture are available.

(3) An intravenous insulin pump may be necessary to control blood glucose concentration.

(4) Surgical debridement to drain pus and abscess cavities and to remove all necrotic and infected tissues. Deep tissue swabs should be sent to the laboratory. If necrosis has developed in a digit, a ray amputation to remove the toe and part of its associated metatarsal is necessary and is usually very successful in the neuropathic foot with intact circulation.

Footwear

Redistribution of weight bearing forces on vulnerable parts of the foot can be achieved by special footwear.

To treat deep indolent ulcers, total contact plaster casts which conform to all the contours of the foot, thereby reducing shear forces on the plantar surface, may be used. Great care must be taken, especially with the fitting of plasters, to prevent chafing and subsequent ulcer formation elsewhere on the foot or ankle.

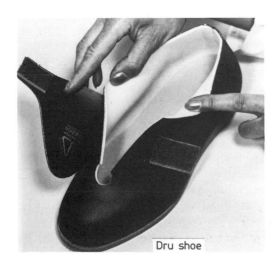

Dru shoe

Moulded insoles made from substances with energy absorbing properties such as plastozote and microcellular rubber are suitable for long term redistribution of weight bearing forces.

Special shoes to accommodate the shape of the foot and moulded insoles are often necessary. In cases of severe deformity shoes may be constructed individually for the patient. However, in most patients, extra depth "stock" shoes will usually suffice.

The neuropathic joint (Charcot's joint)

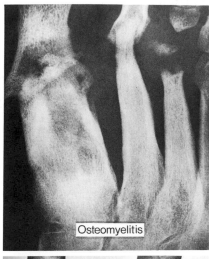

Osteomyelitis

Charcot joints

Loss of pain sensation together with possible rarefaction of the bones of the neuropathic foot may have serious consequences: abnormal mechanical stresses usually prevented by pain may occur, and the susceptible bones are then damaged by relatively minor trauma. Patients present with a hot swollen foot, sometimes aching, and the appearances are often mistaken for infection. Injury may have occurred days or weeks earlier or may not even have been noticed. Sometimes Charcot changes develop after minor amputations which change the normal weight bearing stress. Radiographs at this stage are normal, but bony damage appears and develops rapidly during the following weeks, leading to gross deformity of the foot. The destructive process does not continue indefinitely but stops after weeks or months. Bony changes are most often seen at the tarsometatarsal region of the foot, but they occur also at the ankle or at the metatarsophalangeal region. Changes at other sites are rare.

Early diagnosis is essential. The initial presentation of unilateral warmth and swelling in a neuropathic foot is extremely suggestive of a developing Charcot's joint. Bone scans are more sensitive indicators of new bone formation than radiography and should be used to confirm the diagnosis.

Management initially comprises rest, ideally bed rest or use of non-weight bearing crutches, until the oedema and local warmth have resolved. Alternatively, the foot can be immobilised in a well moulded total contact plaster cast which is initially non-weight bearing. Immobilisation is continued until bony repair is complete, usually in two to three months. In long term management special shoes and insoles should be fitted to accommodate deformity and prevent ulceration, which is the major hazard of the Charcot foot.

Neuropathic oedema

> Neuropathic oedema is associated with severe peripheral neuropathy

Neuropathic oedema consists of swelling of the feet and lower legs associated with severe peripheral neuropathy: it is extremely uncommon. The pathogenesis may be related to vasomotor changes and arteriovenous shunting. Ephedrine 30 mg three times a day has been shown to be useful by reducing peripheral blood flow and increasing sodium excretion.

The neuroischaemic foot

Rest pain

Pain relief with opiates may be necessary in patients with neuroischaemic foot. Paravertebral lumbar block has been disappointing in promoting healing of ulceration, but occasionally rest pain is ameliorated.

Ulceration and gangrene

If the ulcer is small and shallow and not limb threatening medical management is indicated, including eradication of infection, relief of pain, diuretic treatment of peripheral oedema (often associated with congestive cardiac failure), prescription of accomodative footwear, and regular chiropodial debridement of the ulcer.

If the ulcer does not respond to medical treatment, or if gangrene, sepsis, cellulitis, or abscess is present then admission to hospital is indicated and arteriography performed with a view to angioplasty or arterial reconstruction, or both. Infrapopliteal angioplasty or distal bypass to the tibial or peroneal vessels are now well established procedures and important for limb salvage in the diabetic foot.

Amputation of the toe is usually unsuccessful in the neuroischaemic foot (in contrast to the neuropathic foot) unless the foot can be revascularised. If this is not possible, then the necrotic toe should be allowed to autoamputate. Below knee amputation is indicated for rampant infection, extensive tissue destruction, or intractable rest pain in a limb in which reconstruction has not been possible or has failed.

Features and complications of the neuropathic and neuroischaemic foot

Neuropathic	Neuroischaemic
Features	
Bounding pulses	Absent pulses
Diminished sensation	Sensation variable
Complications	
Callosities	Rest pain/pink foot
Painless ulceration	Painful ulceration
Digital necrosis	Gangrene
Charcot's joint	
Neuropathic oedema	

Preventing foot disease: the diabetic foot clinic

Many foot problems can be prevented, so all diabetic patients should be aware of the problem of foot disease. We try to issue every patient with a postcard containing the simplest instructions.

A good chiropodist must be available for diabetic patients. Ill fitting shoes are the cause of many problems. New shoes should always be broken in by wearing them initially for only short periods. If the foot is in any way misshapen—for example, from bunions, hammer toes, Charcot deformities, or as a result of surgery—shoes must be specially made to fit. It is a great advantage if a shoe fitter attends the chiropody clinic: it is possible to make simple shoes fit on the spot (Dru shoes for example) while awaiting delivery of more elaborate fitted shoes made in a workshop.

It is vital that there is close liaison between the chiropodist, orthotist, nurse, physician, and surgeon in the care of the diabetic foot. The diabetic foot clinic is probably the optimum forum for provision of intensive chiropody, close surveillance and prompt treatment of foot infection, and for the provision of specially constructed shoes.

Care of your feet

DO

Wash feet daily with mild soap and warm water

Check feet daily

Seek urgent treatment of any problems

See a chiropodist regularly

Wear sensible shoes

DON'T

Use corn cures

Use hot water bottles

Walk barefoot (except children and adolescents)

Cut corns or callosities

Treat foot problems yourself

Danger signs

- Check your feet every morning
- Come to the clinic *immediately* if you notice:
  Swelling
  Colour change of a nail, toe, or part of a foot
  Pain or throbbing
  Thick hard skin or corns
  Breaks in the skin, including cracks, blisters, or sores

Footwear

For everyday use, especially when on your feet for long periods:
- Wear a lace-up shoe, with plenty of room for the toes, and either flat or low heeled
- Do not wear slip-ons or court shoes, except for special occasions
- Don't wear slippers at home

Neuropathy and the hands

Diabetic neuropathy rarely causes symptoms in the hands, and when it does the disease is already advanced in the feet and legs. Numbness and clumsiness of the fingers are thus very unusual and usually due to some other neurological disorder. Impairment of sensation is, however, often enough to prevent blind diabetic patients from reading Braille.

Paraesthesiae and numbness in the fingers, especially at night, are usually due to carpal tunnel syndrome, which is also common in non-diabetic people. It is easily and effectively relieved by a minor operation performed under local anaesthetic without admission to hospital.

Interosseous muscle wasting, especially of the first dorsal interosseous, is often seen. It is usually due to ulnar nerve compression at the elbow, and typical sensory defects in the fourth and fifth fingers are detectable. It causes little disability and there is no satisfactory treatment. Patients are advised not to lean on their elbows too much, thereby avoiding further damage to the ulnar nerve.

I thank Mrs A Foster, chiropodist, for help with this chapter.

Features of neuropathy of the hands

- Inability to read Braille
- Carpal tunnel compression
- Ulnar nerve compression

DIABETIC NEUROPATHY—II: AUTONOMIC NEUROPATHY

Clinical features of autonomic neuropathy

Gastrointestinal
  Diarrhoea
  Gastroparesis

Cardiovascular
  Postural hypotension
  Persistent tachycardia
  High foot blood flow
  Vascular medial calcification

Genitourinary
  Impotence
  Neurogenic bladder

Sweating
  Gustatory sweating
  Dry feet

Respiratory
  Depressed cough reflex
  Respiratory arrests
  ? Deaths from respiratory arrests

Diffuse damage to both parasympathetic and sympathetic nerves, probably developing in that order, is common in diabetic patients with diffuse peripheral neuropathy. Fortunately the disabling symptoms which result are not common, and even when they do occur some of them, especially diarrhoea, vomiting, and postural hypotension, are curiously intermittent.

Gastrointestinal system

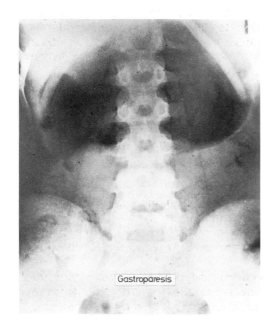

Gastroparesis

Diarrhoea—This is a catastrophic watery diarrhoea with severe nocturnal exacerbations and faecal incontinence, preceded momentarily by characteristic abdominal rumblings. Malabsorption does not normally occur. The symptoms are intermittent, with normal bowel actions in between and sometimes even constipation. These features persist for months or years, sometimes eventually disappearing altogether. The diagnosis is made, firstly, by establishing the presence of peripheral and autonomic neuropathy and, secondly, by excluding other causes of diarrhoea such as coeliac disease. The diarrhoea may be treated with any antidiarrhoeal agent, the best of which is codeine phosphate. Tetracycline in two or three doses of 250 mg has a dramatic effect in about half the cases. Tetracycline should be used only at the onset of an attack.

Gastroparesis—Diminished gastric motility and delayed stomach emptying occur sometimes in diabetic patients with autonomic neuropathy, but they rarely cause symptoms. Intermittent vomiting may occur, and in exceptional cases it may be intractable. Diagnosis is established by the presence of a gastric splash and screening during barium studies; gastroscopy is needed to exclude other gastric disorders. Any antiemetic can be useful, including metoclopramide, domperidone, and cisapride. Erythromycin acting as a motilin agonist has been used but its value has yet to be established.

Cardiovascular system

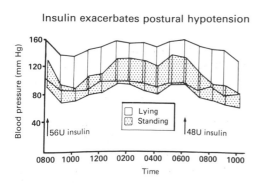

Insulin exacerbates postural hypotension

Postural hypotension (a fall in systolic pressure on standing of more than 30 mm Hg) needs treatment only if symptoms occur and if they are troublesome, which is rare. Patients should stop drugs which might aggravate hypotension (notably tranquillisers, antidepressants, and diuretics), sleep with the head of the bed raised, and wear full length elastic stockings. The best results are obtained from measures which increase plasma volume—namely, a high salt intake and fludrocortisone (increasing the dose slowly to 0.4 mg). Failures are common, and the oedema which results from treatment may be disagreeable. Successful treatment has been reported with indomethacin; a combination of fludrocortisone, flurbiprofen, and ephedrine; the β blocker pindolol; and atrial tachypacing, but these reports have not been confirmed. Midodrine is a new α agonist which is also of some value.

Genitourinary system

> ## Features of impotence
>
> ### Organic impotence
>
> Gradual onset
> Permanent
> Absent nocturnal erection
> Ejaculation often retained
>
> ### Psychogenic impotence
>
> Sudden onset
> Intermittent
> Nocturnal erections occur
> Penile tumescence tests give normal
> results

Impotence is a common problem, but it appears to be commoner in diabetic people. Impotence is, however, most commonly due to psychogenic causes, and it is important that appropriate advice and treatment should be sought from trained counsellors.

Autonomic neuropathy causes erectile impotence, which is permanent and irreversible. Retrograde ejaculation can also occur. The onset of organic impotence in neuropathy is always gradual, progressing over months or even years. Erectile ability fails first, ejaculation declines later. Nocturnal erections are absent in these patients, whereas they are often retained in psychogenic impotence. It is often difficult to distinguish between organic and psychogenic impotence in diabetic patients. The presence of peripheral and autonomic neuropathy makes an organic cause more likely, especially when other autonomic symptoms are present. Newer techniques for examining nocturnal penile tumescence may help in diagnosis.

There is no cure for autonomic impotence. Hormone treatment with testosterone is useless because it serves only to increase libido without improving erectile ability. In many cases, careful explanation of the cause to the affected couples will allay their fears and anxieties.

If active treatment is required there are now three approaches, each of which may succeed, especially when ejaculation is retained:
- Penile injections of papaverine
- Penile condom with applied suction pump
- Rigid penile prosthesis inserted at operation.

Application of these treatments needs specialised counsellors to advise patients on the appropriate treatment and the proper use of the techniques.

Neurogenic bladder—Urinary retention is a serious and usually late complication of autonomic neuropathy. Apart from the discomfort, intractable urinary tract infections may develop. Diagnosis of bladder retention is now simple using ultrasound techniques. Cystoscopy may be needed to exclude other causes of bladder neck obstruction. Treatment is now by self-catheterisation two to three times daily.

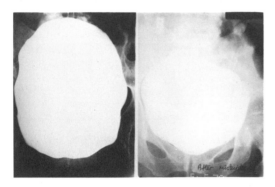

Grossly enlarged bladder before and after micturition.

Other effects

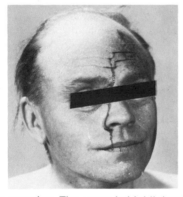

Gustatory sweating. The sweat is highlighted by starch-iodide powder.

Gustatory sweating—Facial sweating (including scalp, neck, and shoulders) which occurs while eating tasty foods, notably cheese, is a common symptom of autonomic neuropathy. When it is very severe it can be treated with anticholinergic agents of which the best is poldine methylsulphate (Nacton).

Respiratory arrests—Transient respiratory arrests occur sometimes if susceptible neuropathic patients are given any agent which depresses respiration, notably anaesthetics. These patients must be monitored carefully even during minor surgery.

Diagnosis of autonomic neuropathy

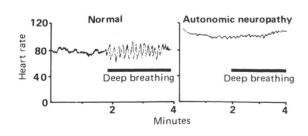

Gustatory sweating is the only symptom which is almost pathognomonic of diabetic autonomic neuropathy. Peripheral neuropathy (at least absent ankle jerks) must be present before the diagnosis can be made. A resting tachycardia, postural hypotension, or a gastric splash may be present.

Loss of heart rate variability during deep breathing is the most reliable and simplest test of autonomic neuropathy. It is best assessed using a cardiotachograph during deep respirations (six breaths per minute) taking average readings during six breaths; it can be performed using an ordinary electrocardiograph during a single deep breath

Diabetic neuropathy—II: autonomic neuropathy

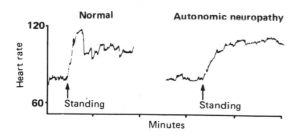

Normal values for autonomic function tests*

	Normal	Abnormal
Heart rate variation (deep breathing) (beats/min)	>15	<10
Increase in heart rate on standing (at 15 seconds) (beats/min)	>15	<12
Heart rate on standing 30:15 ratio	>1.04	<1.00
Valsalva ratio	>1.21	<1.20
Postural systolic pressure fall at 2 min	<10 mm Hg	>30 mm Hg

* These test results decline with age. The figures apply generally in those less than 60 years old.

(five seconds in, 5 seconds out). The heart rate difference (maximum rate during inspiration minus minimum rate during expiration) in the under 55s is always greater than 10. Heart rate increase on standing up should be greater than 12 at 15 seconds, and there should normally be an overshoot as well. The Valsalva manoeuvre can be included among the tests; a mercury sphygmomanometer is used, the patient blowing hard through the empty barrel of a 20 ml syringe to maintain the mercury column at 40 mm for 10 seconds. Maximum heart rate during blowing, followed by minimum heart rate after cessation, are recorded. There should be a bradycardia after cessation of blowing; the ratio of maximum to minimum heart rate is normally greater than 1·21 and clearly abnormal when less than 1·10. Many other sophisticated tests need special equipment.

DIABETIC NEUROPATHY—III:
MONONEUROPATHY AND ACUTE
PAINFUL NEUROPATHIES

Mononeuropathy

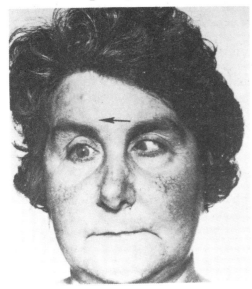

The rapid onset, severity, and eventual resolution of mononeuropathies contrast sharply with the long term nature and irreversibility of diffuse neuropathy. The two forms of neuropathy occur quite independently of each other.

Femoral neuropathy (diabetic amyotrophy)—Pain with or without wasting of one or both thighs is the cardinal feature of this disagreeable condition. The quality of the pain is similar to that in painful peripheral neuropathy, and management is along similar lines. The knee jerk is absent, and sensation on the thigh may be altered or impaired. Other neurological disorders must be considered and excluded. Full recovery within about one year is the rule.

Radiculopathy—Root involvement may cause the characteristic pain in almost any part of the body, notably the trunk.

Cranial nerve palsies—Third and sixth nerve palsies presenting with diplopia of sudden onset are characteristic. Pain behind the eye occurs sometimes in third nerve palsies; the pupil is usually spared, and ptosis does not normally occur. Full examination and careful follow up are needed, but extensive investigation is not normally required. Complete recovery occurs spontaneously in about three months.

Acute painful neuropathy

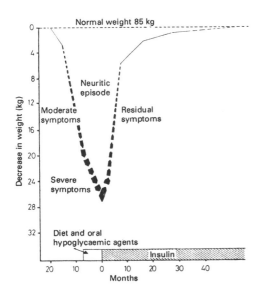

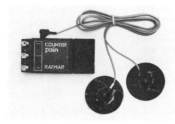

Acute painful neuropathies begin relatively acutely at any stage of diabetes. The acute and persistent pain can be disabling. Distribution of the pain is radicular, affecting either the legs or the abdominal wall over the territory of several adjacent nerve roots. The thighs are affected in patients with femoral neuropathy. Both feet and legs can be affected symmetrically in a stocking distribution. Patients usually recover from these neuropathies in a period of months (up to 18 months). These neuropathies occur independently of the classic sensory or autonomic neuropathy.

The pain causes exceptional distress because it is protracted and unremitting. Constant burning sensations, paraesthesiae, or shooting pains occur, but the most characteristic symptom is a cutaneous hypersensitivity leading to acute discomfort on contact with clothing and bedclothes. The pain leads to insomnia, depression, and weight loss. Patients are so distressed that they may seek several opinions on their condition.

Treatment is difficult, but, above all, the promise that the symptoms always remit eventually may sustain patients during the wretched months of their illness. Diabetic control should be optimal, and insulin should be given if necessary by continuous subcutaneous infusion. Regular analgesics are essential, although drugs of addiction should be avoided. Tricyclic antidepressants are helpful: a useful combination is a preparation containing a phenothiazine (fluphrenazine) with nortryptyline. Carbamazepine can be tried; mexiletene is of doubtful value, as is capsaicin cream. Application of Opsite (a thin adhesive film) can help to alleviate contact discomfort. Vitamins, antiplatelet drugs, aldose reductase inhibitors, and sympathetic blockade are of no value. Electrical nerve stimulators applied to the site of pain may help and patients can take an active part in their treatment.

The photograph of sixth nerve palsy was reproduced, with permission, from *An Atlas of Clinical Neurology* by John D Spillane, published by Oxford University Press. The Raymar nerve stimulator is obtainable from Hodgkinson and Corby, Henley, Oxon.

NEPHROPATHY

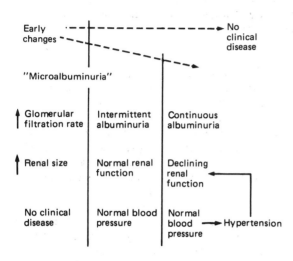

Thirty to forty per cent of all patients with insulin dependent diabetes develop proteinuria, the hallmark of diabetic nephropathy, within 30 years of diagnosis. It usually begins after 15 to 20 years, rarely occurring before five years or after 30 years. The prevalence of nephropathy has decreased during the past 50 years.

White non-insulin dependent diabetic patients are less likely to develop nephropathy than Afro-Caribbean and Asian patients, in whom the incidence of nephropathy is much higher. In non-insulin dependent diabetes proteinuria from nephropathy may be present at the time of diagnosis of diabetes.

End stage renal failure still develops in about 20% of insulin dependent patients diagnosed when less than 30 years old. With the development of transplantation and chronic ambulatory peritoneal dialysis for end stage renal failure the outlook for these patients is relatively good, although problems from coronary artery disease at all stages of nephropathy remains very serious.

Stages of nephropathy

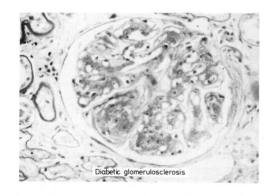

Diabetic glomerulosclerosis

Early physiological changes

At the onset of insulin dependent diabetes there is evidence of hyperfiltration with increased glomerular filtration rate, large kidneys, and large glomeruli. These defects can be reversed by meticulous diabetic control; there is some limited evidence that these changes predispose to the subsequent development of nephropathy.

	Normal (I)	Incipient (II)	Persistent (III)	Clinical (IV)	End stage (V)
Albuminuria (mg/day)	<20	20–300 (Microalbuminuria)	≥300 (up to 15 g/day)	≥300 (up to 15 g/day)	≥300 (can fall)
Glomerular filtration rate (ml/min)	High/normal Hyperfiltration	Normal/high	Normal or decreased	Decreased	Greatly decreased
Serum creatinine (μmol/l)	Normal 60–100	Normal 60–120	High normal 80–120	High 120–400	Very high >400
Blood pressure (mm Hg)	Normal	Slightly increased— 135/85	Increased— 145/95	Increased— 160/100	Increased— 160/100
Clinical signs	None	None	± Oedema, increased blood pressure, may be none	± Oedema, increased blood pressure, may be none	Oedema, increased blood pressure, ureamic symptoms

Course of nephropathy

The natural course of diabetic nephropathy is the progression through five stages from normal renal function to end stage renal failure, as shown in the table. Incipient nephropathy, identified by appearance of microalbuminuria, is the earliest clinical stage and is not associated with significant clinical signs or any changes other than a very small increase in blood pressure. At this stage urine testing (Albustix) will give negative or only trace positive results. Microalbuminuria is detectable by sensitive assays in 24 hour collections or overnight collections, or as a random urinary albumin: creatinine ratio.

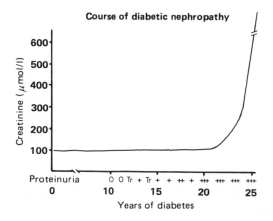

Course of diabetic nephropathy

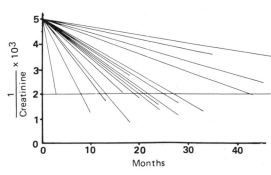

Decline of renal function in 16 patients with nephropathy.

As the disease progresses albuminuria increases, until end stage nephropathy, when it may decrease; there are wide variations in the amount of protein excretion. The glomerular filtration rate shows a progressive decline, which varies considerably between patients and is usefully assessed by calculating the inverse creatinine value (1/serum creatinine concentration) which can be plotted against time and is generally linear.

Blood pressure rises progressively, usually requiring treatment. Nephropathy is commonly asymptomatic until it is advanced, when oedema, breathlessness, and anaemia develop, followed by uraemic symptoms with nausea, vomiting, anorexia, and itching.

Hyperlipidaemia is common in nephropathy, as are other risk factors for vascular disease, including changes in the concentrations of fibrinogen and other clotting factors.

Accompanying problems

Patients with diabetic nephropathy normally have many other complications, the problems increasing as the stage of nephropathy advances. All have retinopathy, often proliferative, and they have a tenfold increased risk of blindness compared with patients without proteinuria. A very high proportion have coronary artery disease, the excess risk of death from this being manyfold higher than in patients without proteinuria. They are also more at risk of peripheral vascular disease, peripheral and autonomic neuropathy, and foot ulceration.

Primary prevention

Poor diabetic control predisposes to the development of nephropathy, although it is not the only factor and there are suggestions of genetic components which may predispose to the disease. Tight control of diabetes early in its course may help to prevent development of nephropathy, although 60–70% of patients will never acquire proteinuria even after many years.

Diagnosis

Investigations in a patient with proteinuria

- Mid-stream urine
- 24 hour urine protein
- Renal ultrasonography
- Blood count
- Erythrocyte sedimentation rate
- Antinuclear factor
- Serum complement
- Serum lipids
- (Renal biopsy only as indicated)

Early detection

Testing urine samples for the presence of protein (Albustix) should be routine practice at every clinic visit. If proteinuria develops it is important to distinguish the onset of nephropathy from other causes of renal disease, especially urinary tract infection and primary renal pathology.

Microalbuminuria can be detected with simple assay techniques and now with rather expensive reagent sticks, which can give false positive results. Positive readings need to be confirmed with 24 hour or overnight urine collections. Screening should at present be limited to patients with insulin dependent diabetes and can be performed every one or two years.

If renal disease evolves gradually over several years in the presence of retinopathy, and there are no unusual features such as haematuria, unequal size kidneys, or a history of urinary tract complaints, then extensive investigation is not necessary. In non-insulin dependent diabetes, however, there is a greater chance of non-diabetic renal disease being present, and renal biopsy may be needed if there are atypical features. In both insulin dependent and non-insulin dependent diabetes the absence of retinopathy should make the doctor suspect other causes of renal failure.

The characteristic pathological lesion is diabetic glomerulosclerosis, including basement membrane thickening, mesangial expansion, and, in the later stages, the classical Kimmelstiel-Wilson nodules, together with hyalinisation of efferent and afferent arteries. Mesangial expansion, which requires an experienced pathologist to interpret, correlates well with renal function.

Treatment

Early nephropathy

At the stage of incipient nephropathy (stage II) improved glycaemic control will reduce the albuminuria and perhaps the likelihood of progression to later stage nephropathy.

Increased blood pressure is often apparently slight, but it should be assessed and treated by using age related blood pressure charts. Once present it should be treated vigorously, aiming at a blood pressure below 140/90 mm Hg or at least less than two standard deviations above the mean for age. Angiotensin converting enzyme inhibitors are now generally the drugs of first choice. Serum creatinine concentration should be measured regularly.

Clinical nephropathy

Once there is established proteinuria of 500 mg/day (corresponding to albuminuria of 300 mg/day or more) improved glycaemic control no longer has a beneficial effect. Treatment of blood pressure, however, is effective in reducing, and in some cases almost stopping, the rate of progression. The aim of treatment should be a gradual reduction of blood pressure using angiotensin converting enzyme inhibitors, diuretics, calcium antagonists, and β blockers. The reduction should not be abrupt, as this may cause a deterioration in renal function, and the drugs must be chosen in the light of the patient's overall condition, complications, and needs. Diuretics are commonly needed to deal with the oedema, which is mainly due to sodium retention.

In patients taking oral hypoglycaemics biguanides should not be used when renal function is impaired because of the danger of lactic acidosis; also long acting, renally excreted sulphonylureas, notably glibenclamide, should not be used because of the risk of accumulation and hypoglycaemia. Drugs such as gliclazide, which are mainly metabolised, are preferable.

Protein restriction may decrease the rate of progression if the dietary intake is cut to about 0·6 g/kg body weight, but this is often difficult to achieve. The best compromise is to ensure that these patients are at least not taking an excessive amount of dietary protein (that is, more than 1 g/kg body weight/day).

Frequent screening for other complications is essential, especially for retinopathy and vascular disease. Serum lipid concentrations should be measured and treatment given when indicated. Smoking should be strongly discouraged.

Approximate expected survival after renal transplantation

	1 year	2 years
Patient survival	90%	80%
Graft survival	70%	60%

End stage renal failure

Patients with end stage renal failure need much time and consideration. Renal support therapy is now available for most of these patients, who should be assessed by a nephrologist once the serum creatinine is 200–300 μmol/l. Transplantation or dialysis is often necessary at a lower serum creatinine concentration in non-diabetic people, often around 450–550 μmol/l. Kidney transplantation is the treatment of choice if the patient has good cardiac function, and full cardiac and peripheral vascular assessments are essential before treatment becomes necessary. If cardiac function is severely compromised then chronic ambulatory peritoneal dialysis is preferable as long term treatment. Haemodialysis is less successful and rarely used as a long term treatment in the UK. More than 75% of patients are alive two years after kidney transplantation, 60–80% of them with satisfactory renal function.

Management of diabetes during transplantation and dialysis

Management of diabetes

At transplantation

1 Continuous intravenous insulin until drips removed

2 Soluble insulin three times a day before meals. Dose about 20% higher than preoperative dose

Then, when diabetes is stable,

3 Soluble insulin three times a day and medium acting insulin at night

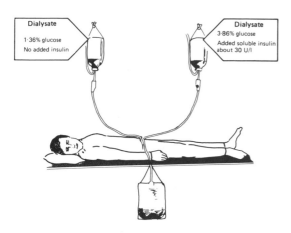

Dialysate

1·36% glucose
No added insulin

Dialysate

3·86% glucose
Added soluble insulin
about 30 U/l

At transplantation—Continuous intravenous insulin infusion is always used, with soluble insulin diluted in physiological saline at 1 U/ml. Infusion rates vary considerably, usually in the range 2 to 20 U/h; during high dose steroid treatment the higher infusion rates are often needed. Intravenous insulin infusion is continued until drips have been taken down and the patient can eat. Soluble insulin is then given subcutaneously three times daily before meals, with an optional fourth dose at midnight if required. The daily dose is started about 20% above the pretransplant dose and adjustments thereafter are made by trial and error. Once reasonable stability has been achieved twice daily insulin is resumed, usually with a mixture of short and medium acting insulins.

During peritoneal dialysis with solutions of low glucose content (usually 1·36% glucose) no adjustment to the normal insulin regimen is needed. Dialysates of high glucose contents can, however, severely disrupt diabetes and additional insulin is needed. During continuous ambulatory peritoneal dialysis insulin can be administered entirely from the dialysis bags: soluble insulin is added to each bag, initially using the existing total daily dose in divided amounts, often giving less at night. The dose may eventually be quite different from that given subcutaneously. The technique is very satisfactory and excellent control can be achieved without hypoglycaemia. Patients whose technique is poor, and who are thus liable to peritonitis, should not be given intraperitoneal insulin.

Rejection—High doses of steroids always upset diabetic control within a few hours. This problem may be anticipated by increasing the first insulin dose after steroids have been given. Intravenous insulin infusion (about 4 U/h) for a few hours as a supplement to the normal subcutaneous insulin is almost always needed until the administration of methylprednisolone has been completed.

Non-diabetic renal disease

Renal arteriosclerosis can occur in patients with hypertension and peripheral vascular disease. Full renal assessment is necessary to distinguish it from diabetic nephropathy

Some patients, especially those with non-insulin dependent diabetes, develop unrelated non-diabetic renal disorders. Clues to their presence have been given above, but renal arteriosclerosis should be particularly mentioned. This is most common in non-insulin dependent patients with hypertension and peripheral vascular disease. Full renal assessment including ultrasonography is essential, although renal arteriography is often required to confirm or exclude the diagnosis. The distinction is vital as angiotensin converting enzyme inhibitors may provoke considerable deterioration in renal function or even precipitate acute renal failure. Glomerulonephritis and other renal disorders can occur in diabetic patients and require renal biopsy for diagnosis and treatment in their own right.

Urinary tract infections

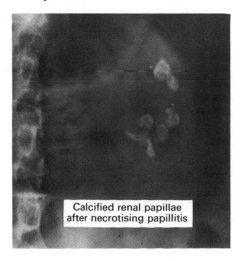

Calcified renal papillae
after necrotising papillitis

Urinary tract infections occur in diabetic people with the same frequency as in non-diabetic people, but they are sometimes exceptionally severe and may cause the renal papillae to slough—necrotising papillitis. Infection is particularly troublesome in the rare patient with urinary retention from neurogenic bladder. Diabetic control is easily disturbed by urinary infection, as with any infection, and must be regained quickly, with insulin if necessary, while the infection is treated with antibiotics.

Pyelonephritis with septicaemia is not uncommon in diabetes, with occasional formation of perinephric abscesses. The source of the infection may not be immediately apparent and sometimes patients present in profound shock without an obvious site of infection.

PREGNANCY

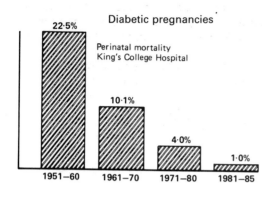

Diabetic pregnancies

22·5%

Perinatal mortality
King's College Hospital

10·1%

4·0%

1·0%

1951–60   1961–70   1971–80   1981–85

Fifty years ago about a quarter of diabetic pregnancies ended in fetal death. Now almost all are successful. This remarkable improvement is due to major developments in obstetric, diabetic, and paediatric care. Major congenital malformations, however, still occur more commonly than in normal pregnancies.

Management of established insulin dependent patients

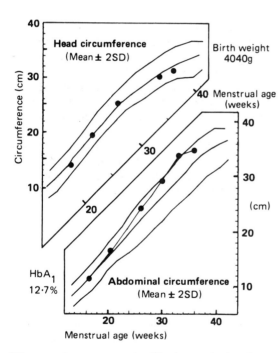

Ultrasound measurement of fetal growth showing excessive increase of abdominal girth, indicating delivery of a large baby.

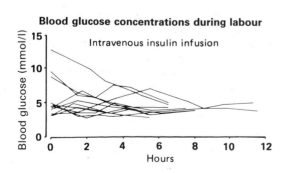

Blood glucose concentrations during labour

Intravenous insulin infusion

Education of diabetic women of child bearing age is important: they should be advised that if they plan a pregnancy their diabetic control should be optimal (haemoglobin A_1 should preferably be < 10%) at the time of conception and during the early weeks of pregnancy. This advice is very important for all diabetic women and especially those who have had a previous catastrophe in pregnancy. Optimal control early in pregnancy may reduce the incidence of congenital malformations. The clinic notes of young diabetic women are therefore tagged and clearly marked after advice has been given to avoid repetition.

Pregnant diabetic women should report to their doctor or clinic as early as possible in pregnancy and be referred without delay, preferably to a centre where joint diabetic, obstetric, and paediatric care is available. Team care of this kind is probably the most important factor responsible for the improved prognosis for these pregnancies. An early ultrasound examination establishes the exact gestational age and detects major fetal abnormalities.

Diabetic control should be optimal throughout pregnancy; if it is not admission to hospital, even for short spells, should be arranged without delay. Home blood glucose monitoring is the ideal technique for most pregnant diabetic women, while others should perform three or four urine tests each day. Twice or thrice daily insulin injections are needed, and patients should be taught how to adjust their own insulin doses. The dose of insulin needed often increases substantially during pregnancy, sometimes to twice or three times the usual dose. Blood glucose values should be maintained as near normal as possible and should preferably be kept below 6 to 7 mmol/l, though postprandial values may sometimes be a little higher. Good blood glucose control is quite easily achieved in pregnancy, and continuous subcutaneous insulin infusion is rarely needed.

Most patients should be admitted for a short period before planned delivery or for a longer period if there are any problems. Fetal growth is carefully monitored by regular ultrasound measurements; fetal heart rate and its beat-to-beat variation are monitored regularly by an instantaneous heart rate meter. Delivery is planned to take place as near to term as possible, unless there are medical or obstetric indications for earlier induction; the aim is for vaginal delivery whenever possible.

Labour

Regimen	Blood glucose	Infusion rate
	<3 mmol/l	½ U/h
	3–6 mmol/l	1 U/h
	>6 mmol/l	2 U/h

If dexamethasone is used in premature labour insulin must be infused at the same time to avoid severe hyperglycaemia

Insulin and glucose are given by intravenous infusion for all vaginal deliveries as follows:

Intravenous dextrose (5%)—1 litre every 8 hours delivered at a steady rate.

Intravenous insulin—Soluble insulin diluted in physiological saline (1 unit insulin per 1 ml saline) and administered from a syringe by infusion pump at about 1 U/h (usual range 0·5–2 U/h). If very low infusion rates are used the insulin concentration may be halved.

Blood glucose concentrations should be maintained at 3 to 6 mmol/l. Insulin infusion is continued until the patient can restart her normal meals: the *prepregnancy* insulin dose is then restarted; otherwise severe hypoglycaemia will occur.

Premature labour—Because of the hazards of premature labour attempts may be made to promote fetal lung maturity by giving dexamethasone. This causes severe hyperglycaemia unless an intravenous insulin infusion is started at the same time as the administration of dexamethasone. Large doses of insulin may be needed.

Caesarean section—Insulin infusion is always used, as described in the section on management during surgery (see chapter on diabetic emergencies).

The neonate

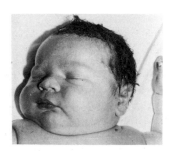

"... they convey the distinct impression of having had such a surfeit of food and fluid pressed on them by an insistent hostess that they desire only peace so that they can recover from their excesses."

J W Farquhar (*Arch Dis Child* 1959;**34**:76)

The babies of diabetic mothers are still larger than normal; however, they no longer need routine care in special care baby units unless there are specific reasons. Respiratory distress syndrome is now rarely seen in these infants. Blood glucose concentrations should be checked regularly, especially in jittery babies, because hypoglycaemia is still commoner than in the infants of non-diabetic mothers. Polycythaemia, hyperbilirubinaemia, and hypocalcaemia are also commoner among these infants.

Breast feeding is encouraged in diabetic mothers as in non-diabetic mothers. The mothers' diet should be increased by about 50 g of carbohydrate daily and ample fluids taken. The insulin dose is not usually affected if these measures are followed.

Diabetic complications

Diabetic women with established nephropathy normally should be advised against pregnancy

Retinopathy—Fundi should be examined routinely at the beginning and end of pregnancy. If retinopathy is present at the beginning then more frequent examination is needed because occasionally progression is rapid during the course of pregnancy. If proliferative changes are present photocoagulation should be performed urgently.

Nephropathy—Patients with proteinuria from nephropathy can expect problems during pregnancy with an increased risk of fetal loss. When this is considered, together with the knowledge that the mother may need dialysis or transplantation within a few years, many of these patients should be advised to avoid pregnancy.

Patients with nephropathy who become pregnant can expect to become hypertensive, and fetal growth may be delayed. Hypertension is treated with methyldopa, hydralazine, or occasionally labetalol or nifedipine; thiazides should not be used in pregnancy, though frusemide can be given if a diuretic is needed. Angiotensin converting enzyme inhibitors are contraindicated because of adverse effects on the fetus. Early delivery of a premature infant is often required, but with good neonatal care most infants survive. Protracted inpatient care in a specialised unit is needed for a successful outcome.

Diabetes discovered during pregnancy (gestational diabetes)

Fetal size and mortality in women discovered to have even mild diabetes during pregnancy are still greater than normal. These patients should therefore be given the same careful treatment as established diabetic patients.

Indications for glucose tolerance test

- Glycosuria:
    random 1–2%
    random glycosuria traces twice or
        more
    fasting glycosuria
- Fasting blood glucose >5·6 mmol/l
- Random postprandial blood glucose after two hours or more >6·1 mmol/l
- Previous gestational or latent diabetes

Diagnosis

Routine blood glucose measurements are made in every pregnant woman between 26 and 30 weeks.

- A random blood glucose concentration >11·1 mmol/l is diagnostic of diabetes (see p 1)
- A fasting blood glucose concentration >8·0 mmol/l is diagnostic of diabetes (see p 1)
- If the fasting blood glucose concentration is >5·6 mmol/l perform a glucose tolerance test
- If a random postprandial blood glucose measurement taken after two hours or more is >6·1 mmol/l perform a glucose tolerance test.

All women who have previously had gestational diabetes should have a glucose tolerance test between 26 and 30 weeks unless there are indications to perform it sooner. *A two hour blood glucose concentration greater than 9·0 mmol/l establishes the diagnosis of gestational diabetes.*

Where routine blood glucose measurements cannot be performed in normal pregnancies, urine glucose testing should be undertaken. If one fasting or two postprandial samples give positive results a glucose tolerance test should be performed.

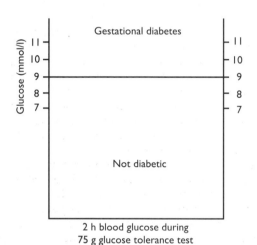

2 h blood glucose during
75 g glucose tolerance test

Treatment

Gestational diabetes is initially treated by diet alone. If control deteriorates (that is, preprandial blood glucose concentration regularly exceeds 6–7 mmol/l) insulin should be used. Oral hypoglycaemics are not usually used, though there is no evidence that they are harmful.

Postpartum

A glucose tolerance test should be repeated six weeks after delivery. Most values return to normal; these women, however, have about a 50% risk of developing non-insulin dependent diabetes later in life. An annual check of blood glucose concentration is desirable, and they should be advised to avoid excessive weight gain. Those patients who remain diabetic after pregnancy should be treated in the usual way.

Contraception and diabetes

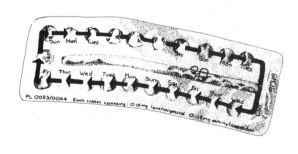

Contraceptive advice to diabetic women is, in general, the same as for non-diabetic women. Use of the contraceptive pill makes little difference to diabetic control, although a small increase in insulin dose may be needed. The combined low dose oestrogen-progestogen or progestogen only pill may be used. Care is required if oral contraceptives are given to women who have had gestational diabetes, since they can cause deterioration of glucose tolerance and development of diabetes. In these circumstances oral contraceptives are probably best avoided, but if they are used urine tests and blood glucose measurements should be performed after about three months. There is no sound evidence that oral contraceptives cause more problems in diabetic women than in non-diabetic women; contraindications are the same in both groups. Nevertheless, doubts about their safety have been expressed, and barrier contraceptive methods may be preferred.

Support at the joint diabetic antenatal clinic is given by Dr Marjorie Doddridge, Mr K Nicolaides, and Dr H Gamsu and I acknowledge their help in preparing the first figure.

ORGANISATION OF DIABETIC CARE: SHARED CARE SCHEMES

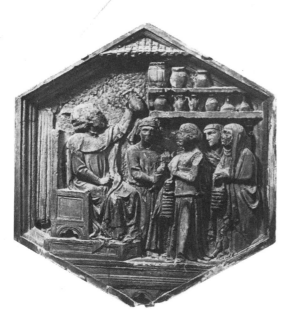

Doctor's surgery: tile from the Campanile in Florence by Andrea Pisano, about 1340.

Care of diabetic patients requires enthusiasm and organisation. There are various ways of undertaking it, but without interest and motivation, none will succeed.

It is best to bring diabetic patients together into properly organised clinics, whether in general practice or in hospital, so that they can benefit from the wide range of special services needed for their proper care. The best strategy for achieving optimal treatment is a system of shared care, in which a close liaison is forged between general practitioners and hospital specialists. Diabetes shared care schemes are very advanced in many parts of the UK and set a model for other specialties as they represent the same time both efficient treatment and ideal links between hospitals and the community.

A shared care scheme aims to deliver the best care to patients. In order to do so there must be an efficient two way flow of information about patients, and the shared experience of a dedicated staff. Dissemination of expertise among all those concerned is essential. Schemes require constant nurturing and audit and should ideally be performed with research projects in order to bring about innovation and renewal.

Staff

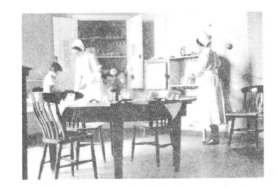

Diabetic kitchen, King's College Hospital, 1935.

Nurses—The backbone of diabetes care systems is provided by well trained, dedicated nurses, ranging from those primarily concerned with the general practitioner clinic; through those involved with the community, who also act as a link between the general practitioner and the hospital; and those predominantly committed to the hospital service. They should work as a coherent team with responsibilities ranging from giving direct care and advice to individual patients to organising educational programmes both for diabetic patients and for all the nursing and medical staff who care for them. Thus health visitors, district nurses, practice nurses, and specialist nurse practitioners will all be members of this team. At least some of them should have specialist training and be involved with the British Diabetic Association. While it is clear that nursing expertise can now provide for many of the patients' needs, shared care schemes must involve nurses and doctors working closely together, and schemes in which nurses are caring for patients in isolation should not be encouraged.

Dieticians are integral members of the team and, like the nursing staff, can offer their services both in hospitals and the community.

Organisation of diabetic care: shared care schemes

<table>
<tr><td>

The diabetes care team

- Diabetes physician
- General practitioners
- Diabetes nurses
- Dietitian
- Chiropodist
- Opthalmologist
- Obstetrician
- Orthopaedic surgeon
- Vascular surgeon
- Renal physician
- Paediatrician

</td></tr>
</table>

Chiropodists are needed both for routine foot care and preventive measures on the one hand and for treating foot disorders, chiefly in hospital, on the other. There are serious shortages of chiropodists throughout the UK; better provision of high quality chiropody would reduce both morbidity and amputation rates among diabetic patients.

Doctors—A wide range of properly coordinated doctors is needed to cover the whole range of problems arising in diabetes. These include not only hospital diabetes specialists; ideally the team should also work with a dedicated ophthalmologist, obstetrician, orthopaedic surgeon, vascular surgeon, renal physician, and paediatrician and preferably a neurologist as well. In the future hospital contracts should include sessions dedicated to diabetes in these specialties. General practitioners undertaking diabetic care need a range of medical and organisational skills (as defined in the British Diabetic Association's *Guidelines for the Development and Integration of GP Care of Diabetes with Hospital Based Systems*).

Diabetes services

<table>
<tr><td>

St Vincent Declaration

A joint European initiative between the WHO and the International Diabetes Federation (IDF) resulted in the publication of the St Vincent Declaration in 1989, which calls for targets for improving the outlook for diabetic patients. The recommendations include:
- Reducing new blindness due to diabetes by a third or more
- Reducing numbers of people entering end stage diabetic renal failure by at least a third
- Reducing by a half the rate of limb amputations for diabetic gangrene
- Cutting morbidity and mortality from coronary heart disease in diabetic patients by vigorous programmes of risk reduction
- Achieving pregnancy outcome in diabetic women that approximates that of non-diabetic women

</td></tr>
</table>

A complex range of services is needed for comprehensive diabetes care. This is provided between general practice and hospital systems in the joint shared care scheme, as follows:

- Diagnosis, education, and treatment of new patients
- Routine care for long term patients with ongoing education
- Screening aimed at preventing complications
- Education programmes for individual patients, groups of patients, and all nurses and doctors involved in care of diabetic patients
- Provision of expertise, literature, and teaching aids in a resource centre, usually based at the hospital department
- Emergency access for patients and doctors (a direct telephone line is essential)
- Specialist services, all of which should ideally be conducted jointly with individual consultants in the relevant specialties:
  Retinopathy clinic
  Antenatal clinic
  Children/adolescent clinics
  Foot clinics (including peripheral vascular disease)
  Renal clinic
  Neuropathy clinic.

Operation of shared care schemes

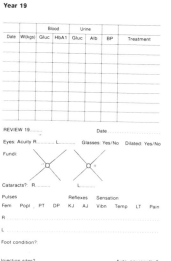

Page from a diabetic record card for patients.

Most general practices are likely to become involved with diabetes shared care, and it follows that most patients will in future be seen in these schemes. Care of diabetic patients is thus divided between (a) the general practitioner and practice nurse; (b) nurse education for individuals and groups (in general practice or hospitals); and (c) hospital specialist services.

Thus symptomless, well controlled patients without complications will attend general practice services most and hospitals least, while those with increasing symptoms and inadequate control will attend hospital services most. Patients who should normally attend hospital for all or at least part of their care are: pregnant women; children and adolescents; those with diabetic complications; and most insulin dependent patients.

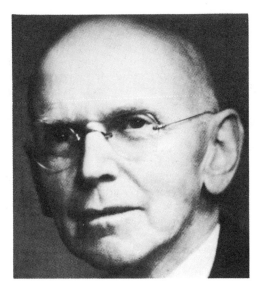

Elliott P Joslin, 1869–1962.

Obviously the requirements for diabetes care will vary from one geographical area to another, but anyone who undertakes the care of diabetic patients must heed the words of the late Dr Elliott P Joslin: "To retain his patient for 20 years he must shun proprietary remedies as the devil does holy water, continually seek for new knowledge as eagerly as the diabetic grasps for life, but ever sift the wheat from the chaff remembering that faithful treatment in season and out of season is rewarded."

The photograph of a diabetic kitchen was reproduced by permission of the British Diabetic Association and that of Elliott P Joslin by Lea and Febiger.

PRACTICAL PROBLEMS

Employment and hobbies

Hypoglycaemia is the major hazard for any insulin treated diabetic patient

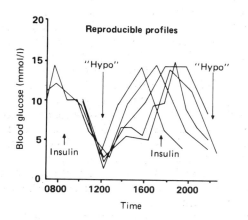

Reproducible profiles

Most of the problems of diabetic people in society result from the ever present possibility of hypoglycaemia in insulin treated patients. Although this hazard is small in many individuals, it is an unacceptable risk in some circumstances. The guiding principle in making the difficult assessments for employment or hobbies is whether the risk of confusion during hypoglycaemia affects only the individual or whether it also places the safety of others at risk.

Individual firms and industries have generally established their own regulations about the suitability of diabetic people for particular jobs. If candidates for employment are rejected unreasonably solely on account of diabetes they may appeal. Diabetic people are not normally accepted by the armed forces, the police, the merchant navy, or the fire brigade. Shift work, especially night shift work, should be avoided if possible by those taking insulin, but suitable diabetic people can certainly make appropriate adjustments and many may successfully cope with such work.

Diabetic people treated by diet alone or with oral hypoglycaemic tablets who are otherwise fit should be permitted to undertake any occupation or hobby. Their risk of hypoglycaemia is negligible.

Some diabetic people who find difficulty in obtaining work may find it useful to apply for registration as a disabled person. Sometimes this makes it easier for diabetic people to find work and they can remove themselves from the disabled register at any time.

Driving

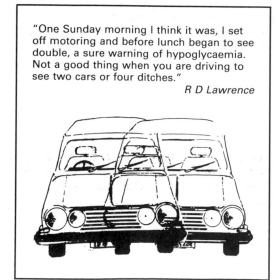

"One Sunday morning I think it was, I set off motoring and before lunch began to see double, a sure warning of hypoglycaemia. Not a good thing when you are driving to see two cars or four ditches."

R D Lawrence

Diabetic people who are otherwise physically fit and not suffering from blackouts are normally allowed to hold ordinary driving licences. The law demands that all patients whether treated by tablets or insulin should inform the Driver and Vehicle Licensing Agency, Swansea. If applying for a licence for the first time the appropriate declaration must be made on the application form. It is helpful to indicate whether or not insulin is being used. Driving licences are granted for three years and are reissued (at no extra fee) subject to a satisfactory medical report.

Healthy diabetic people treated with diet or tablets are normally allowed to hold both heavy goods vehicle and public service vehicle licences. Diabetic patients receiving insulin treatment may not hold public service or heavy goods vehicle licences because of the serious potential consequences of hypoglycaemia, no matter how small the risk may be to any individual diabetic patient.

All insulin treated diabetic people who drive should always keep a supply of sugar in their cars. They should try not to drive if they are late for a meal, when the danger of hypoglycaemia is great. If they experience warning symptoms of hypoglycaemia they should stop, switch off the ignition, and preferably leave the car, since they may otherwise be open to a charge of driving under the influence of drugs (insulin).

Insurance and pension

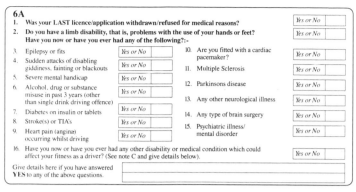

Driving licence application form.

Driving insurance with a normal premium will usually be issued, subject to a satisfactory medical report. Life assurance premiums are often raised by amounts which depend on the result of a medical examination. It is worth looking for the "best buy." Sickness and holiday insurance premiums are often higher than normal. The British Diabetic Association offers helpful advice on insurance.

Small supplementary pensions are available to help diabetic people with the increased cost of food for their diets. Patients who are registered blind are eligible for supplementary pensions.

Travel

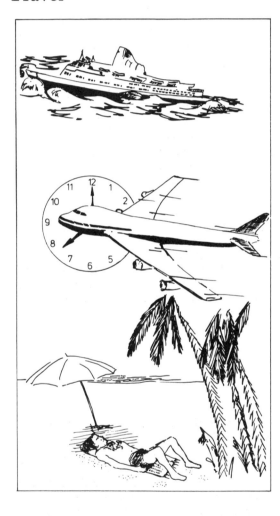

Diabetic control is easily upset by the rigours of travelling. Diabetic people should therefore undertake regular urine (or blood) tests and adjust diet and insulin if necessary. Some of the following circumstances present special problems.

Sea sickness—Diabetic people may use the same anti-seasickness tablets as non-diabetic people: these drugs do not change diabetic control. They tend to cause drowsiness, so it is best not to drive. If vomiting occurs insulin should be continued without fail and the situation dealt with as described in the chapter on diabetic emergencies.

Time changes on long distance air travel will inevitably make diabetic control difficult for a few days. It is best to change the time of each injection by two or three hours: there should be no difficulty in adjusting to a six hour change of clock time within 24 hours. If the time between injections is long a small supplementary injection of soluble insulin (perhaps 4 or 8 units) may be needed if urine or blood tests deteriorate. Conversely, if the time between injections is short a small temporary decrease of dose may be wise. Urine or blood should be tested every four to six hours during the period of changeover.

Physical activity—More insulin may be needed if the diabetic person decides to be much less active when on holiday, or vice versa. Dietary indiscretions may also play havoc with control.

Breakage or loss of equipment—Diabetic people should take ample supplies of syringes, insulin, needles, and testing equipment. The equipment in current use and that for emergency use is best kept in separate places. Soluble and isophane insulins may be obtained in most countries.

Storage of insulin—In a temperature climate insulin will keep for some months at room temperature. (Injections sting less if the insulin is not chilled.) Refrigeration, however, would be wise for prolonged visits to tropical climates. It is also recommended if stocks are kept at home for long periods. Insulin should never be deep frozen and should not be left in the luggage hold of an aircraft, where it may freeze.

Vaccination and inoculation are quite suitable for diabetic people and should be given for the same indications as for non-diabetic people.

Dental treatment

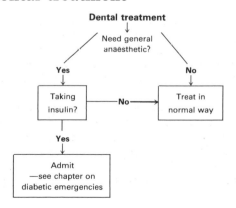

Diabetic people may receive dental treatment in the normal way and without any special arrangements, except in the case of insulin treated patients needing a general anaesthetic, when a short admission to hospital is the wisest course.

INDEX